W9-BJK-936

LAKE VILLA DISTRICT LIBRARY
(847)356-7711 www.lvdl.org

3 1981 00645 0476

OMG
IT'S TWINS!

ALISON PERRY

Ver LAKE VILLA DISTRICT LIBRARY
847.356.7711   www.lvdl.org

To my three daughters.
Without you all, this book wouldn't be possible.

1

Vermilion, an imprint of Ebury Publishing,
20 Vauxhall Bridge Road,
London SW1V 2SA

Vermilion is part of the Penguin Random House group of companies
whose addresses can be found at global.penguinrandomhouse.com

Penguin
Random House
UK

Copyright © Alison Perry 2021
Design © Nikki Dupin at Studio Nic&Lou 2021
Illustrations © Veronica Dearly 2021

Alison Perry has asserted her right to be identified as the author of this
Work in accordance with the Copyright, Designs and Patents Act 1988

First published by Vermilion in 2021

www.penguin.co.uk

A CIP catalogue record for this book is available from the British Library

ISBN 9781785043130

Commissioning Editor: Samantha Jackson
Editors: Emma Owen, Leah Feltham, Justine Taylor & Lindsay Kaubi
Designer: Nikki Dupin at Studio Nic&Lou
Illustrator: Veronica Dearly

Printed and bound in Great Britain by Clays Ltd, Elcograf S.p.A.

The authorised representative in the EEA is Penguin Random House Ireland,
Morrison Chambers, 32 Nassau Street, Dublin D02 YH68.

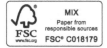

MIX
Paper from
responsible sources
FSC® C018179

Penguin Random House is committed to a
sustainable future for our business, our readers
and our planet. This book is made from Forest
Stewardship Council® certified paper.

The information in this book has been compiled as general guidance on the specific subjects addressed.
It is not a substitute and not to be relied on for medical, healthcare or pharmaceutical professional
advice. Please consult your GP before changing, stopping or starting any medical treatment. So far as the
author is aware the information given is correct and up to date as at December 2020. Practice, laws and
regulations all change and the reader should obtain up to date professional advice on any such issues. The
author and publishers disclaim, as far as the law allows, any liability arising directly or indirectly from the
use or misuse of the information contained in this book.

CONTENTS

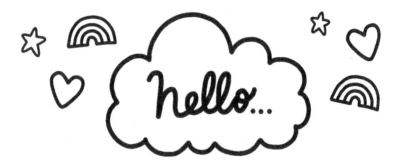

You're pregnant! And it's TWINS.

I've got a whole bunch of questions for you. How are you feeling? Was it a shock when you found out there are TWO humans growing inside you? Have you had any morning sickness? Have you been extra tired? OK, I'll stop with the questions because let's face it, there's a good chance you've been getting a lot of those from friends and family if this is news you've already shared with them. And you don't need to hear them from me!

I'm Alison and as a mum of twin girls (they are somewhere between the baby and toddler stage as I'm writing this) I've learned a thing or two about giving birth to and raising twins. In this book I'm going to share my experiences and I'm also going to speak to lots of people who are experts – from midwives and doulas to psychotherapists and nutritionists – who will impart their amazing wisdom. And I'm going to ask lots of twin mums to share their experiences with you, because if there's one thing I've learned about motherhood, it's that there is no one right way to do anything. Anyone who says 'Guys! I've cracked this mum stuff, and if you follow my step-by-step plan, you'll crack it too!' should be swiftly avoided. There are lots of approaches, lots of ways to tackle a problem, lots of solutions, and what works for one baby might not work for another. (Which makes having twins even more fun because working out what they need from you is double the fun!)

So what's the point of this book, then? When I was pregnant with my twins, I asked around the twin mums I knew: 'OK, what's the twin book that I need to buy?' and the response involved tumbleweed, a shrug of the shoulders and a few suggestions of this book or that book, but most of them came back to say they didn't think a brilliant twin book existed. How can this be? I wondered. We need a book that guides us through all of the emotional ups and downs of twin pregnancy, preparing for the birth, going through the birth, and then preparing for the fourth trimester (that's the first three months after giving birth!) because it's a total roller coaster!

We need a book that holds our hand through it all, offers emotional support and gives us practical answers in a non-judgemental way. We need to hear stories from the mums who have been there and advice from the experts who know their stuff. We need a book that will put your mind at ease and help you with that feeling of overwhelm.

So, here is that book! *OMG It's Twins!* is designed to be dipped in and out of (because we're busy people, right? And once you have those babies, you probably won't want to sit down to wade through a wordy book). There are tips, ideas, some interactive pages for you to fill in, and above all else, lots of supportive and helpful stuff to guide you through the next few months.

You can totally nail this twin thing, and this is the start of a big adventure . . .

Love,

Alison

MUM OF THREE - ONE BIG SINGLETON AND TWO LITTLE TWINS x

MINI PREGNANCY JOURNAL

I'M FEELING:

I'M WEARING: I'M EATING:

I'M **EXCITED** ABOUT: I'M *nervous* ABOUT:

PREGNANCY

It's easy to think that the challenges of being a twin mum start when you give birth but a twin pregnancy can be as demanding as a Hollywood film star. You might sail through the next few months feeling fine or you might find yourself experiencing some major pregnancy symptoms (see page 32 for those).

Whatever your twin pregnancy is like, this section should answer any questions you've got and give you an insight into some of the things that other pregnant twins mums have experienced.

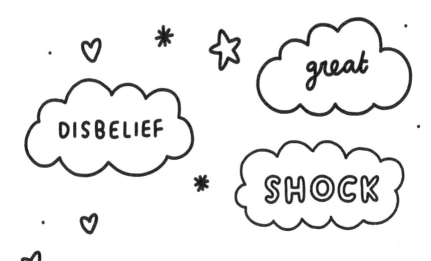

WHEN I WAS TOLD I WAS HAVING TWINS, I FELT...

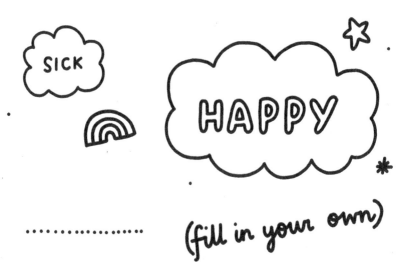

.... (fill in your own)

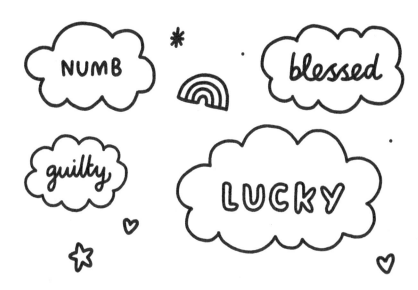

NUMB

blessed

guilty

LUCKY

(COLOUR IN THE ONES YOU FELT)

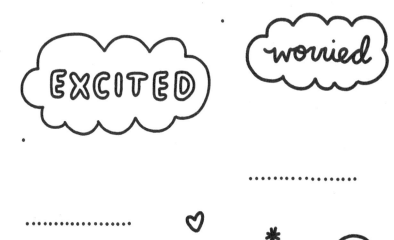

EXCITED

worried

9

Chapter 1

The moment you find out (OMG!)

I'll never forget the day we were told we were having twins. We were at our 12-week scan and as I popped (hoisted) myself up onto the hospital bed, the sonographer asked if this was our first scan. I explained that – no – we'd had a scan at six weeks. This pregnancy was the result of IVF after years of secondary infertility, so when we saw those two blue lines on the pregnancy test, our fertility clinic had booked us in for a six-week viability scan.

At the six-week scan, like so many couples, we were hoping and praying for a heartbeat, and for everything to look as it should. When the consultant scanning me pointed out the sac and the heartbeat of the one baby in my uterus and told me everything looked good, we left the clinic feeling utter relief.

And we spent the next six weeks planning for our one baby.

At the 12-week scan, the sonographer squeezed the cold ultrasound gel onto my tummy. 'Great! You've had a scan already, so you know it's just the one baby then?' she chatted away.

We laughed. 'Yes! Just the one baby.'

The sonographer started scanning me and very quickly looked confused before sharing the news that we were, in fact, having . . .

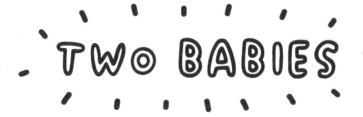

At that moment, my husband and I dissolved into uncontrollable giggles.

Discovering you're pregnant with twins can be a massive shock. There's no right or wrong way to react to the news. Chances are you've spent the past few weeks feeling excited about having one baby growing inside you – and probably feeling a little worried about getting to that important first scan – and suddenly, you're thrown a huge curveball. You're digesting the news that there are two babies growing inside you.

You might have had a long journey to get to the point of being pregnant – suffered loss, disappointment – you might be feeling anxious about the pregnancy progressing safely, or worried about the effects a twin pregnancy could have on your body and mind, you might simply be unable to get your head around the practicalities of looking after two babies at once!

It's completely normal to feel a whole range of emotions. I felt excited, nervous, utterly blessed and terrified all at once. Like a mojito of feelings, all mixed together in a big shiny cocktail shaker.

Lying there, being scanned in the hospital room, my head was spinning and I couldn't stop laughing. You know that nervous laughter you did as a child when you were being told off by a teacher and no matter how sternly they looked at you, you just couldn't stop? Like that. I kept apologising to the sonographer because my abdomen was shaking from the laughter, which must have been making it tricky for her to carry on scanning me.

Afterwards, we had a short wait in the waiting room. 'I can't believe it,' I said to my husband, 'TWINS!' Suddenly I was aware that he might be very much not OK with this news. Even though I was the one sat there with two humans growing inside me, this was a lot for both of us to take in. We chatted about how we were feeling – in shock, a bit numb, but OK – and before I knew it, we were in another small, dark room waiting to speak to a consultant who worked on the hospital's specialist twin team.

She was a very serious lady (well, I guess she has a serious job) and she explained that we were expecting monochorionic diamniotic – MCDA – twins, which meant nothing to me at the time, but I googled it and saw it meant identical twins that share a placenta but have their own amniotic sacs. This meant it was a high-risk pregnancy. The consultant ran through all of the risks involved and said that from week 16 of pregnancy I'd be scanned every two weeks.

We had another wait in the hospital waiting room, and sitting there I felt overwhelmed with emotion – more than anything, I felt worried for these two little babies and just hoped they'd make it all the way to being born safely. I already knew a bit about Twin to Twin Transfusion Syndrome (TTTS) – the main risk to MCDA twins like mine – and I knew it was a potentially life-threatening condition to one, or both, of the babies. (There's more info about TTTS on page 44, but in a nutshell, it's when twins sharing a placenta don't receive blood flow evenly – one twin gets more blood than the other and it can be dangerous for both of them.)

Inside me, this fear was swirling around with excitement at the idea of having twins – I mean, they're a miracle, right? We had a seven-year-old daughter already and I'd always secretly wanted three children, so now we were jumping the queue, from one child to three! Just like that!

Mixed into it all I felt anxious about how we'd cope with two small babies. I'd suffered from postnatal depression seven years earlier when my eldest was little, and I was already worried that it would resurface, especially with two babies to look after this time. (Two babies!)

So how did I deal with the fear? I did what I often do when I'm feeling scared and I turned to humour: I WhatsApped my friends, saying, 'At my 12-week scan. Guess what?!' and sent them a photo of Arnold Schwarzenegger and Danny DeVito from the 1988 Hollywood movie *Twins*.

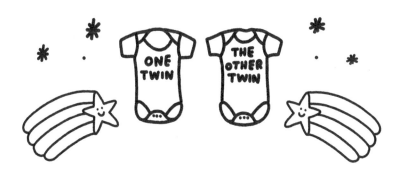

Twin types, explained . . .

There are a few different types of twins and you'll see them referred to throughout this book, and in your medical appointments.

* **Dichorionic diamniotic twins (DCDA)**
  Each twin has their own separate placenta with its own separate inner membrane (amnion) and outer membrane (chorion). All non-identical twins are DCDA, and one third of identical twins are DCDA.

* **Monochorionic diamniotic twins (MCDA)**
  These twins share one placenta with a single outer membrane and two inner membranes. Two-thirds of identical twins are MCDA.

* **Monochorionic monoamniotic twins (MCMA)**
  These twins share one placenta and share both the inner and outer membranes. One in 100 identical twins are MCMA.

I'd bet that every mum who's told she is expecting twins will feel a bit differently to the next – when you consider just how many human emotions there are (a study found that there are 27) and how we can often feel varying degrees of different emotions at the same time it's not surprising.

Here's our first expert, Anna Mathur, talking about some of the negative thoughts you might be having . . .

<u>5 THINGS</u> you might experience (*& why it's OK to feel this stuff*)

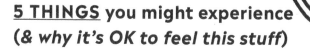

Anna Mathur (@annamathur), psychotherapist and mum of three

1 STRESS

When we receive news we weren't expecting, the body's nervous system produces adrenaline and cortisol, and the heart might speed up – it's the stress response in the body. That can continue for a little while afterwards, so you might just be going about your day and then suddenly, the reality hits you: 'Oh my gosh, I'm going to have twins!' It's completely normal to feel this way. The important thing to know is that feelings come and go like waves. There's often a real fear that if we let ourselves feel something negative, we'll feel that way forever, we don't always trust these difficult feelings to be transient. But try to view emotions like waves – you might have times of feeling excited and times of feeling nervous – and if you engage in those nerves, it doesn't mean that you'll feel like that for the rest of your pregnancy. Let it be. Observe your feelings and sit with them. Then allow those feelings to wash away again.

2 FEAR

It's normal to feel terrified. And not surprising when you think about the way people talk about having twins – it's often in a negative way. When someone's pregnant with one baby, people might joke about the size of the bump and say, 'Are you sure you haven't got two in there?' which isn't the most positive of messages. And as a pregnant twin mum, you might hear the phrase 'Double trouble!' These messages and the assumptions we have in our own minds about having twins shape how we respond and react to the news of being pregnant with twins. Of course you're going to feel terrified.

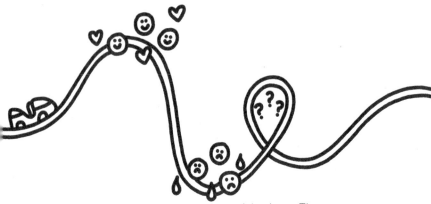

Of course you're going to feel nervous. Of course you might even have thoughts like, 'How the heck am I going to deal with this? What if I don't want this?' That's all part of the process. Allow someone else to help you process those thoughts and help to rationalise them. Find a friend or two who have been supportive in the past and who are able to journey with you through all the different emotions that are coming and discuss how you're feeling.

3 ANXIETY

Anxiety can kick in when we start to overthink things. It's normally based around being worried or tense about the future – we start building stories in our head of how things might go and we think about potentially

tricky times. Then our nervous system gets involved, and that's when we can start to feel anxious and panicky. It's a very normal reaction to have when you're given the news that you're expecting twins.

Try writing a journal where you reflect on your feelings at the end of each day. (See page 20 for a great practical exercise.) The better we get to know ourselves and our feelings and needs, the more confident we will be in tending to them, and then those negative feelings are more likely to wash away.

4 GRIEF

It might sound odd to say that you might feel grief, but the news that you're expecting twins has changed everything. So often, we project to the future. You

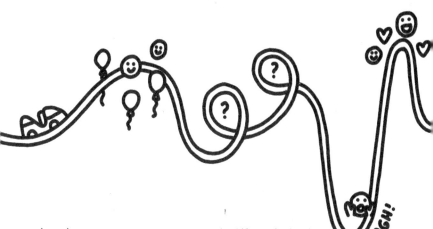

imagine you are pregnant. You imagine you have one baby. You imagine what life is going to be like that with that one baby. If you've spent months or years imagining your life will be one way and your whole idea of your future is shaped around that and that suddenly changes, a shift has to happen. So there can be grief involved, and for some, it might be a more pertinent grief than for others. But we can grieve a dream, we can grieve an expectation. That's a natural feeling to have. It's OK to feel a sense of grief, even if you're happy about the news you're expecting twins.

5 GUILT

You might feel guilty for having negative feelings towards the news you're pregnant with twins.

And if you feel guilt, an important question to ask yourself is: Have you actually done something wrong? If someone took you up in front of the court and said, 'What's your crime?' and you said, 'Oh, my crime is that I'm pregnant with twins and I'm finding it really scary. And I'm finding it hard come to terms with the fact that I'm going to have to juggle two babies and I don't know how the heck I'm going to do that,' are they going to send you to prison? No! So why punish yourself for feeling incredibly normal emotions? Negative feelings are not reflective of your love and your capacity to love your babies. It's OK to feel two conflicting emotions, even if those two things feel completely contradictory.

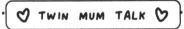

♡ TWIN MUM TALK ♡

'I was terrified to be told I was having twins'

FIONA, MUM OF A FIVE-YEAR-OLD DAUGHTER
AND IDENTICAL TWIN BOYS, AGED THREE

———————

As soon as they started to scan me at my 12-week scan, I saw two babies on the screen straightaway. I burst into tears and jumped up to standing. Thirteen years earlier I'd been told by a medium that I'd have identical twins. I didn't believe her at the time, partly because I'm an identical twin and the chances of an identical twin having identical twins are so slim. It was so spooky to be told that she was right – twins! But that wasn't the only reason I was upset. I didn't have the best experience as a twin, growing up. My mum and twin sister both nearly died during the birth and I've carried an awful lot of guilt around knowing that. I also found growing up tough, being compared to my identical twin sister and the fact that my identity was so closely linked to hers. Carrying around all of these issues, I was terrified that history would repeat itself.

The following week I started having therapy to help me through what I was feeling, and it really helped to talk it all out with someone. Something else that made me feel so much better was when – at 16 weeks – I found out I was having boys. It meant that their experience wasn't going to be the same as mine. It was such a relief.

Thankfully the birth went smoothly and although I knew it was going to be hard work, being a twin mum to these little boys, I knew I could do it.

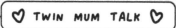
'We've been trying for six years to have a baby & now we're having two!'

CHANTAL, PREGNANT MUM OF NON-IDENTICAL TWINS

When I saw the positive pregnancy test I felt happy but cautious – we'd been through seven rounds of IVF over six years, we'd had a miscarriage and we'd had one pregnancy that ended very sadly with us being told the baby wasn't compatible with life. So staring at those two blue lines on the pregnancy test at 4am one morning, we knew it was just the next hurdle that we'd successfully managed to leap over.

At our first scan it was immediately very obvious to my husband and me that there were two big black circles on the screen. But the sonographer didn't say anything, so I asked, 'Is there a baby there?' and he said, 'Yep, there is!' So then I asked, 'Just the one?' and he said – really casually – 'No! There are two!' We'd spent years not knowing if we were ever going to have one baby and here we were being told we're having two babies. It felt like we'd just won the lottery – twice!

I had so many other feelings too – a really strange mix of emotions. It sounds selfish but I thought, 'Oh, I'm not going to find out what it's like to have a single baby.' And in a weird way, it felt a bit greedy. There are so many couples trying to have one baby and we're having two. Because of my history I'm just praying we get to 37 weeks – every scan I go into I'm a ball of nerves. I can't believe in a few months' time we'll have gone from zero to a complete family!

Anna Mathur's FFN exercise

Something I find helpful when processing big news is thinking about 'FFN' - **Fear**, **Feeling**, **Need**.

* **Fear** - is there anything I'm worried about right now?

* **Feeling** - what am I feeling at the moment?

* **Need** - what do I need? Perhaps it's reassurance? Is it connection with another pregnant twin mum so that I can talk about it with them? Is it a hug? Or do I need to jot down some practical stuff so that if I can get it out of my head and onto paper?

Get a piece of paper, or your journal, and draw three columns with Fear, Feeling, Need at the top. Write down some thoughts under each. Then chat it over with your partner or a family member. Having it written down often makes it easier to process and talk through.

Of course, you might be feeling none of these things - you might just feel pure elation and joy! Don't read this list and feel like you perhaps should be feeling worried or stressed.

'I'm so stressed about the fact I'm not stressed! Why am I not stressed?'

Enjoy the peace you feel with your twin pregnancy news.

IF YOU ONLY DO 3 THINGS

1 Allow yourself to feel unsettled by the news.

2 Write down how you're feeling, each day, to give yourself the chance to process it.

3 Try not to overthink things – you've got a while to think about, and do, what you need to.

Chapter 2

Getting your head around it

It's a lot to get your head around, isn't it? As the news sinks in that you're pregnant with two babies, be kind to yourself. Not only are you growing two new humans inside you (and believe me that can leave you feeling absolutely knackered) but your head is getting used to the idea.

It's OK not to be OK about this, immediately.

You might keep the news a secret or you might be bursting to tell everyone – I broadcast our twin news far and wide – but there's no right or wrong way to react, it's just how you feel about the situation, and everyone's situation is different.

Perhaps keeping it to yourselves for a little while is exactly what you need – a chance to get used to the idea before you share it with others. We'd already told our friends and family that I was pregnant – we did that after our six-week scan – so we were happy to tell everyone: 'SURPRISE, IT'S TWINS!' after our 12-week scan.

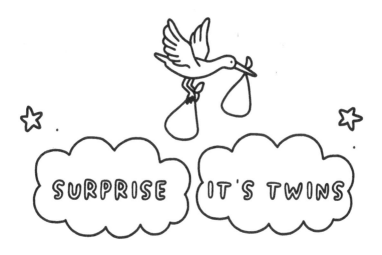

SURPRISE IT'S TWINS

It helped me get used to the idea. Chatting to school mums about it on the school run and seeing everyone's reactions on Facebook made it seem more real to me. If I hadn't had that I might have suspected I'd dreamed the whole scenario.

In fact, I soon found myself telling everyone – 'It's twins!' I called to Sharon the lollipop lady as I crossed the road patting my belly. Seeing her excited reaction made me feel more excited.

Of course not everyone will react with excitement – you might get a look of horror from someone, or they might simply say, 'Good luck with that!' or trot out a well-used cliché like, 'Double trouble!'

Try not to let the reactions of others affect how you're feeling about this. Their reaction often says a lot more about them than you. The great news is, for every person who reacts in a less-than-ideal way two or three will just beam at you with joy.

How people might react	What it actually means	What you could say!
'Rather you than me!'	They would find it hard to cope with two babies and that might be because of their own personal experience, but it has nothing to do with your experience, how you will cope or how you feel.	*'When shall I book you in for babysitting then?'* Often making a joke (even if you're feeling annoyed) is a good way to end the conversation and move on with your day.
'Double trouble!'	They're possibly not sure how to react so they've reached into their brain and said the first thing they associate with twins. They very possibly don't mean it as a negative.	*'Double the cuddles!'*
'Are they natural?'	While it might feel like a super personal question, people so often hear about twins being the result of fertility treatment that I think often this question is blurted out before the person has really thought about what they're asking. Which is essentially: Did you and your partner have sex to conceive or not?	I think light-heartedly brushing this off is a good way to go, so laugh and say something like, *'Ooh, that's a bit of a personal question for the supermarket!'* and then immediately change the subject: *'Did you see that nappies are half price here? I must stock up before the babies arrive!'*

'Other people's reactions were unhelpful'

SARAH, MUM OF NON-IDENTICAL TWINS, AGED TWO

I couldn't believe how many people made negative comments when I found out I was expecting twins. 'Rather you than me!' someone close to me blurted out. 'Double trouble!' spluttered stranger upon stranger as soon as they learned, upon enquiry, that my enormous bump was indeed twins. To be honest, I felt sorry for them; I felt as though they'd truly missed the point. What an incredible privilege to be carrying two babies.

I had my own concerns, of course. Like any expectant parent, I was concerned for their healthy arrival. And I was concerned, once they were born, that I'd be constantly totting up how much time I spent with each twin, how many hugs and kisses I gave each of them. But, now that they're here, like any siblings, they're uniquely different people. They don't need my affection, time and attention split exactly down the middle, they just need me when they need me.

I was warned it would be twice the work. Let me tell you now, if you're expecting twins, in my experience, it's twice the fun. Twice the joy. Double first smiles, first laughs, first tastes of ice cream. And the best part about twins? Well, other than double the love, the best part is that I don't feel guilty or neglectful when I leave them for a few minutes to do something else. They're never alone.

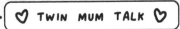

We had a six-month-old baby when we found out we were having twins

KAREN, MUM TO EIGHT-YEAR-OLD IDENTICAL
TWINS AND A NINE-YEAR-OLD DAUGHTER

———

We had a six-month-old baby – my daughter Lily – when we found out I was pregnant with twins. I remember thinking, 'But what are we going to do? We're going to have three babies!' As the news sank in, my mind went to the practicalities – that's just the kind of person I am. We'd recently bought a new car and I remember thinking that we were going to have to sell that because we couldn't fit three car seats in. 'Am I going to be able to get out of the house?' I wondered. 'What buggy can I have for a toddler and twin babies?' But there was also a bit of fear.

We don't have family living close by, so I knew we wouldn't have any day-to-day support and I was worried how we'd manage. We'd always known that we wanted to have children close together – but not that close together! And we didn't expect to have twins! I became obsessed with watching any TV programme about couples with multiples – you know, the shows where they have four, six, eight babies. I'd think, 'OK, if they can do that, I can do this.'

When we told our friends and family, the main reaction was laughter – I think they just couldn't believe that we were having twins so soon after having Lily. The laughter certainly helped lift the mood a bit. And thankfully, my family did end up being around to help when the twins arrived.

If you've got other children, you'll probably be working out when's the best time to share the news. We told our daughter (who was seven at the time) as soon as she got home from school on the day of our scan. We'd already texted a few family members and friends from the hospital and we'd sworn them to secrecy so we could tell her ourselves. 'We had the scan and saw the baby!' I said, as she walked in the door with her dad. I handed her a print-out of the scan, which clearly showed a baby. She gasped and grinned. 'Oh my gosh!' she said. Then I handed her a second scan and said, 'And we saw the other baby too!' After allowing her to look confused for a few seconds, we said, 'It's twins!' Her grin got even bigger. 'Oh my gosh!'

She had always dreamed of having twin sisters, and although we didn't know at that point whether they were girls or boys, she was crossing her fingers firmly for girls.

Questions you ask yourself. . .

In the hours, days and weeks after you discover that you're having twins there are lots of things you might be thinking about. Questions I asked myself included:

* *Will I cope looking after two babies?*
* *Will I be more likely to have postnatal depression?*
* *How big will my bump get?*
* *Do we need to buy two of everything?*
* *Is it possible to breastfeed twins?*
* *How will I be able to tell my identical twins apart?*
* *How will my daughter feel going from being an only child (and getting all our attention) to being one of three?*

Clinical psychologist Dr Emma Svanberg says that writing down all of these questions and worries can really help us. Here's what she has to say . . .

3 WAYS to process the news that you're having twins

Dr Emma Svanberg (@mumologist), clinical psychologist

1 Try to embrace the positives *and* the negatives

When it comes to twin pregnancies there are risks that it is worth being aware of, but, as with all pregnancies, there are also many unknowns and lots we could feel anxious about. If you have become pregnant after a long journey of fertility struggles that anxiety can be even more heightened. Anxiety is often a physiological reaction to a psychological threat – our body in 'fight, flight or freeze mode', prepared to deal with the threat coming our way. Really, what this brings out in us is primal – a fear for the safety of our children. It's common to try to distract ourselves from our anxiety but instead it can be helpful to turn towards it and think about what we are perceiving as threatening. How likely is it to actually happen? We can feel guilt and shame about feeling anything but joy when it comes to pregnancy and parenthood, but ambivalence – feeling conflicting feelings at the same time – is part and parcel of pregnancy and parenthood.

You're facing a big life change, it would be strange if you didn't have some mixed feelings! And some parts of the experience are tough, and a twin pregnancy can take a lot out of you physically. So let yourself feel all the feelings, and talk about them so that they don't become something shameful.

2 Brain dump the practical stuff

It can be overwhelming when your mind is racing with all the practical elements of having twins. They are valid worries, so facing them with your partner can be really helpful. Try sitting down together and getting it all on paper, thinking about what you'll need - not just practically but physically and emotionally too. I find Mind Maps (see page 30) a really useful way of getting worries down on paper.

You can brain dump absolutely everything that you are worried about, without judgement, and then begin thinking of possible solutions. One of the great things about being a twin mum is that people are more accepting of your need for support, so make sure that one of those solutions is to get as much help as possible.

3 Redefine *your* expectations

It can be useful to think about what you're expecting of yourself. What images do you have in your mind about how life is going to be? What are you doing in those images? What does that say about what you're expecting of yourself? If you really question it, are those expectations realistic? What ideas about being a 'good mum' are you bringing to this experience? And how many of them do you think will add pressure and raise anxiety?

It's amazing when you really drill down into it just how much you might be subconsciously demanding of yourself. Talking to other twin mums can be so useful, just to do a reality check.

DRAW A MIND MAP

Get your concerns down on paper by creating a **MIND MAP**.

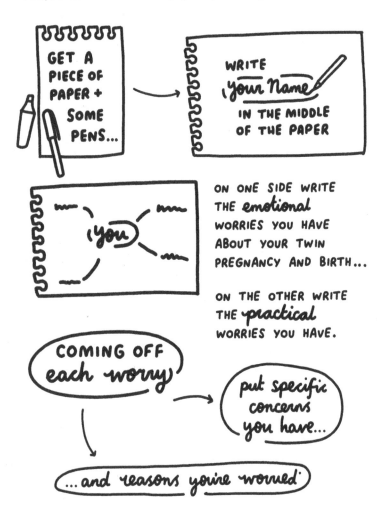

GET A PIECE OF PAPER + SOME PENS...

WRITE *your Name* IN THE MIDDLE OF THE PAPER

ON ONE SIDE WRITE THE *emotional* WORRIES YOU HAVE ABOUT YOUR TWIN PREGNANCY AND BIRTH...

ON THE OTHER WRITE THE *practical* WORRIES YOU HAVE.

COMING OFF *each worry*

put specific concerns you have...

...and reasons you're worried

IF YOU ONLY DO 3 THINGS

1 Don't take other people's negative reactions to heart.

2 When you worry about something, ask yourself: How likely is it to actually happen?

3 Do a **MIND MAP** (*see left*) of your worries.

Chapter 3

What *will* your twin pregnancy be like?

So you've got your head around this. It's happening. You're having twins. But what's your twin pregnancy going to be like? The truth is: no one knows. It's different for every mum and for every pregnancy – I know mums who've got two sets of twins and their pregnancies were very different.

By now you've possibly had a bunch of first-trimester symptoms – nausea, indigestion, extreme tiredness and feeling dizzy or light-headed are all very common. And they can be awful! It sometimes feels like because something happens to lots of us, it gets brushed under the carpet and dismissed as being 'just one of those things'.

So let me be the one to say this to you:

'Normal' first-trimester twin pregnancy symptoms SUCK. And they often seep into the second trimester too, so you might be at 15, 16, 17 weeks and still feeling terrible. Not fair, right?

With a twin pregnancy, you're more likely to suffer from morning sickness because – as midwife Layla Toomer explains on page 40 – you've got two placentas or one big placenta, which means more pregnancy hormones buzzing about, doing their thing. In fact, a twin pregnancy can mean 30–50 per cent higher levels of human chorionic gonadotropin – hCG – and it's this hormone that's thought to cause morning sickness.

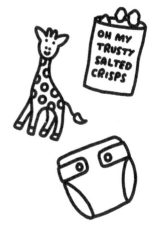

I spent around six or seven weeks feeling nauseous and exhausted – some days were tougher than others and saw me being sick a few times throughout the day. I knew that the morning sickness (worst name for a condition ever, right? If only it just happened in the mornings . . .) was linked to blood-sugar levels, so I tried to keep them stable by regularly grazing on any bland food that I could stomach. Don't judge me, but I ate a lot of bowls of Coco Pops and packets of ready salted Hula Hoops in those weeks!

I felt super tired all the time, so I took it really easy. I didn't feel up to making plans and seeing friends, or doing lots of fun outings with my daughter, and I spent a lot of time on the sofa, working at my laptop or watching Netflix. I felt incredibly grateful to be a freelancer who could push back a few deadlines – it was a far cry from my last pregnancy when I'd had to drag my grey-faced, nauseous self to the office every day, pretend to my colleagues that I felt fine (because I hadn't told them I was pregnant yet) and then drag my sorry ass back home where I'd fall asleep on the sofa. If that's your reality with this twin pregnancy, then let me tell you: I know how hard it is. I found that telling my boss, at around seven weeks helped because at least if she knew why I was being quiet in meetings/ nibbling gingernut biscuits/ saying no to post-work drinks it made things easier.

But I appreciate that not everyone has an understanding boss and there might be lots of political and personal reasons why you don't want people at work to know.

During all of that though, I felt a whole heap of GUILT. I felt guilty for not being able to spend lots of quality time with my daughter (**Her:** 'Can we play a game?' **Me:** 'Mummy's not feeling very well. Can you see if Daddy will play with you?'). But I also felt guilty about not feeling 100 per cent filled with joy every day. We'd had two rounds of IVF and other fertility treatment – five years of trying and failing – to get to this pregnancy. Shouldn't I be feeling totally blessed from the moment I wake up to the minute I fall asleep?

The reality is that I'm not sure it's even possible to feel that way, even without first-trimester pregnancy symptoms making you feel pants. So I gave myself a good talking to and reminded myself that it's OK to feel sorry for yourself during pregnancy. It's possible to feel terrible and still, deep-down, be over-the-moon happy that you're pregnant.

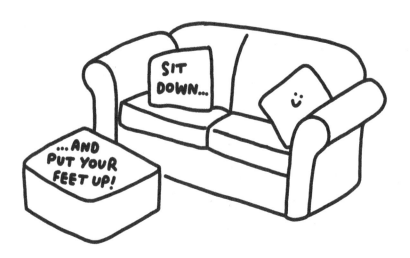

10 THINGS that might happen to your body during your twin pregnancy (*and how to handle them*)

1 MORNING SICKNESS

Want a miracle cure for morning sickness? I'm really sorry to be the one to break the news to you . . . it doesn't exist. You'd think, by now, it would. But things that can ease the symptoms a bit include eating little and often (keeping blood-sugar levels stable seems to help), resting, eating carbs but avoiding foods high in fat and/or sugar, having a small snack before you get out of bed in the morning, drinking ginger tea and wearing acupressure wristbands.

2 EXHAUSTION

Changes in hormone levels, a growing placenta (or two) and your babies' major organs being formed can all contribute to you feeling utterly zapped of energy in the first trimester. It's common to have a bit more energy in the second trimester, and then often by the third trimester – especially with a twin pregnancy – insomnia, strange dreams and carrying around the weight of that extra baby can leave you feeling fatigued. Listen to your body – rest when you can, catch up on sleep when you can and eat a healthy diet to give you some energy (see p. 62 for more on nutrition).

3 STRETCH MARKS

Lots of us are already familiar with stretch marks (streak-like marks on the skin that can be pink, red, purple or brown in colour) before pregnancy, but some of us get a lot of them during pregnancy, and even more so with a twin pregnancy. They affect eight in 10 pregnant women and they're caused by the skin stretching and the middle layer of the skin (the dermis) breaking in places. With a twin pregnancy, you're

LISTEN TO YOUR BODY. REST WHEN YOU CAN

likely to grow a bigger bump, so your skin has further to stretch, which means stretch marks are even more likely to appear. Using creams and oils to help your skin's elasticity is said to help your skin stretch and avoid stretch marks appearing, so it's a good idea to moisturise your tummy area from the very start of your pregnancy. (It's also a really nice pampering routine to get into, and looking after yourself like this will help your mental wellbeing too!)

4 CHANGES TO YOUR BREASTS

Some women say that their breasts feeling different is the first sign that they are pregnant. The changing hormone levels during pregnancy can make your breasts feel tender (a bit like just before a period) and they're likely to grow in size due to the fat layer in your breasts thickening, the production of more milk glands and increased blood flow to the area. All of this is your body preparing for breastfeeding. It can be a good idea to buy new bras (many women find they become broader across the back too, because of the rib cage expanding to make room for the baby) and contrary to popular belief, they don't have to be non-wired. Wear whatever is comfy! If you're keen to get value out of your new bras, some maternity bras double up as nursing bras, which means you can wear them once the babies have arrived. You might also find that your breasts leak colostrum (the thick creamy milk that you produce before making breastmilk). If this happens, pop breast pads in your bra, to absorb the milk. Don't worry though, if you don't notice any changes to your breasts – lots of us don't, and that's normal too.

5 BACKACHE

This is such a common pregnancy woe and it's caused by your ligaments softening to prepare your body for labour, which puts extra pressure on your lower back and pelvis. Gentle stretches (see page 71 for more) can really help and so can wearing flat shoes, avoiding heavy lifting and keeping your back straight and well-supported when you're sitting. If the back pain is particularly bad, speak to your midwife or GP.

6 HEADACHES

These are particularly common in the first trimester so make sure you're drinking plenty of water and getting plenty of rest. If you get a headache, you can take paracetamol but avoid other painkillers like ibuprofen. Headaches can sometimes be a sign of a serious pregnancy condition like pre-eclampsia so speak to your midwife straight away if you develop a severe headache, have problems with vision, develop a pain just below your ribs, suffer from vomiting or have a sudden increase in swelling of your face, hands, feet or ankles.

7 PILES

One of the less glamorous symptoms of pregnancy, piles (aka haemorrhoids) are swellings containing enlarged blood vessels inside or around your bottom. Pregnancy hormones (yes, those hormones again!) make your veins relax, which can cause the piles. To ease the symptoms eat high-fibre foods and drink plenty of water (see page 63 for more on what's advised during a twin pregnancy), avoid standing for long stretches of time, and do gentle exercise. You can push any piles that are sticking out of your bottom back in (be gentle and use a lubricating jelly if you need to).

8 VARICOSE VEINS

During a twin pregnancy, we produce more blood to support the babies, which puts extra strain on our veins and can cause them to swell. The increase in hormones also causes the vein walls to relax and the growing uterus can put pressure on veins in the pelvic area. If you suffer from varicose veins, try to avoid standing for long periods of time, try not to cross your legs when you sit down, put your feet up as much as you can (best advice ever, no?) and do gentle exercise (see page 71 for more on this) to help your circulation.

9 HEARTBURN

Indigestion can be caused by hormonal changes and the uterus putting pressure on the stomach. With twin pregnancies, it can be more common because of the extra pressure from two growing babies. The burning sensation in your chest during or just after eating can be very unpleasant. Some things you can do to alleviate this are sitting upright while you eat, eating little and often and cutting down on rich or spicy food. You can also buy over-the-counter indigestion remedies which are handy to keep in your bag

10 SWOLLEN FEET AND ANKLES

A sudden increase in swelling can be a sign of pre-eclampsia (see page 43 for more) but a gradual increase in swelling is very normal and usually not harmful. It's caused by your body retaining more water than usual, and it can be worse when the weather is warm or you've been standing up for long periods of time. To help ease the swelling, don't stand up for long, get lots of rest, put your feet up, do gentle exercise and drink lots of water. In warmer months, wear sandals that you can loosen when you need to. In colder months, comfy shoes like trainers that you can loosen off when your feet swell up are handy.

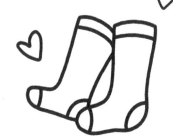

'I was diagnosed with pre-eclampsia and gave birth at 32 weeks '

KATIE, MUM TO IDENTICAL TWINS, AGE SIX

My pregnancy didn't exactly go smoothly – at around 22 weeks, one of my twins started to show extra amniotic fluid during scans, which can be a sign of Twin to Twin Transfusion developing. At 29 weeks, I had a premature labour scare and I was admitted to hospital for four days. Only a few weeks later, at 32 weeks, I had some pretty significant swelling in my legs and feet. I started to feel nauseous and was retching a lot. I also couldn't wee more than the tiniest drop, even though I felt like I needed to. The babies were moving much less than usual and I'd started contracting again. I rang triage who told me to come in.

Tests quickly showed that my blood pressure was very high and my urine contained protein. While they waited for my blood test results I was moved to the delivery suite – all the signs were pointing towards pre-eclampsia, which might mean an immediate delivery. I felt panicked at the thought of the girls arriving so early. My blood tests showed that my kidneys were not functioning well at all and around the same time, it became clear that one of the babies was becoming distressed.

From that point, things moved very quickly and I was taken into theatre for an emergency C-section. I felt quite worried and like it was all out of my control, but I just wanted my girls to be born safely. They're now six and super bright little girls – you'd never know they were born so early!

4 things you should know about a twin pregnancy

Midwife and twin specialist Layla Toomer

1 You're more likely to get ANY pregnancy complication

Because you've got two babies in there, two placentas – or one big placenta – and additional pregnancy hormones, you are more likely to get all of the complications that are associated with pregnancy. That's why it's really important that twin mums are seen regularly by a midwife for blood pressure checks and urine analysis.

2 If you've got monochorionic twins, whether or not you develop TTTS is completely out of your control

It's purely down to the placenta. There's nothing you can do or avoid to change the course of what will happen, so try not worry about it too much. But do be aware of the potential symptoms in between your scans – be aware of how you're feeling and how your tummy feels. If you think something has changed, I urge you to see your midwife quickly. Some pregnant mums worry about wasting their midwife's time, so they say nothing until their next appointment, but we'd much rather see you, scan you and either tell you everything is fine or pick up on an issue quickly.

3 Listen to your body and rest if you need to

Twin mums often struggle because they're carrying around more weight. If you've got a couple of good-sized babies, a good-sized placenta or two placentas, and fluid, then often by around 28–30 weeks, a twin mum is at the equivalent size to a full-term singleton pregnancy. And you've still got a few weeks to go, after that. So it's important to rest whenever you feel tired.

Be open-minded about when you might need to go on maternity leave

Often one of the first things a pregnant twin mum asks me is: 'When would you suggest I go on maternity leave?' It's really difficult to answer because everyone is different and it depends on what your job is like and how your pregnancy is progressing. You might want to go on maternity leave a bit sooner than singleton pregnant mums, particularly if you've got a physical job. It's highly unlikely that you're going to reach your due date with a twin pregnancy, and it's likely you'll be having your babies early, so I always think it's quite nice to have a little bit of maternity leave beforehand to get ready for the babies. I often suggest thinking about starting maternity leave at around 34 weeks. But if you're struggling, then consider leaving work earlier than that.

How to ace your antenatal appointments

✱ Before each appointment it's a good idea to make a list of any questions or concerns you have (I'd make notes on my phone and then I knew I wouldn't forget them!).

✱ Remember to take your hospital notes with you – and take some water and a snack in case you have a long wait!

✱ Don't feel silly mentioning any symptom and don't feel rushed – your midwife is there to set your mind at rest or investigate anything you're feeling.

✱ Remember, your employer is legally obliged to give you time off for all of your antenatal appointments.

Conditions you *might* suffer from during your twin pregnancy

While there's more chance of you developing a pregnancy condition, the good news is that you'll have more antenatal appointments than mums with a regular singleton pregnancy. So there's going to be lots of opportunities to ask midwives and consultants about all of these possible complications, and to chat about how you're feeling. Here's what to keep an eye out for ...

Condition	What is it?	What can I do to deal with it?
Hyperemesis gravidarum	Extreme nausea and sickness caused by increased pregnancy hormones.	Rest as much as you can and avoid any nausea triggers (smells, sights, moving images)
Gestational diabetes	When your body doesn't make enough insulin, which results in high blood-sugar levels. Urine tests at antenatal check-ups should spot this.	Your midwife should give you diet and exercise advice, which might help, and if not, you might be prescribed a medicine like metformin.
Obstetric cholestasis	Extreme itching caused by an issue with the liver, which results in bile salts building up in your blood.	Advice includes wearing loose, non-synthetic clothes, using aqueous cream and you may be prescribed ursodeoxycholic acid (UDCA) to reduce bile acids.

Pre-eclampsia	A condition that causes high blood pressure, headaches and swelling of the feet, face and hands and might require bed rest or early delivery.	Pre-eclampsia can only be cured by giving birth to the babies, but you may be prescribed medication to deal with high blood pressure.
HELLP Syndrome	A rare liver and blood clotting disorder, which is a variant of pre-eclampsia and may require early delivery.	Like pre-eclampsia, the only way to treat HELLP Syndrome is to deliver the babies.
Symphysis pubis dysfunction (SPD)	The extra weight of two babies and increased hormones can cause pelvic pain.	Wearing a pelvic support belt can help. Try to be as active as possible but rest when you can.
Anaemia	When your body doesn't have enough red blood cells or haemoglobin to carry oxygen around your body in the blood.	Take iron supplements (with orange juice, which helps the absorption), eat dark green leafy veg, pulses and meat.
Pre-term labour	The average length of a twin pregnancy is 36.4 weeks, but it's possible to go into labour prematurely.	Stay active during your pregnancy, look after your mental wellbeing, avoid smoking, drinking and drugs – these things all contribute towards early labour.

Of course, twin pregnancies bring with them some extra complications and they're often classed as 'high risk'. Being told your pregnancy is high risk and having all of those risks listed at you is never going to fill any pregnant mum with joy and calm. Hearing, 'It's twins! But all of these things might go wrong in the next six months . . .' is a bit like being given the biggest bar of chocolate you've ever seen, while being told in detail about the risks of diabetes, heart disease and obesity. While it's important to be aware of the things that might potentially happen during your twin pregnancy, it's also a good idea to try to think positively. The majority of twin pregnancies go smoothly and result in healthy babies being born.

And that's the goal, right? A boring pregnancy and a run-of-the-mill birth!

Within an hour of finding out we were having twins, we were told that – because our twins were sharing one placenta – I was at risk of Twin to Twin Transfusion Syndrome (TTTS). It was explained to us that from Week 16 I'd have a scan once a fortnight to keep an eye on things. It would have been perfectly reasonable to have flown into a panic at this point. After all, I was being told that my twins might develop a rare but life-threatening condition. But somehow I managed to stay calm. I remember thinking to myself: 'Let's just deal with things as and when they happen.' Thankfully, my husband had a similar view. 'We could walk outside tomorrow and be run over by a bus for all we know,' he said to me. 'We can't sit here worrying about whether that might happen or not . . .' He was right. Me stressing about things that could go wrong in my pregnancy wouldn't make things any less likely to go wrong.

So, from Week 16, off I went to the hospital every two weeks for a scan. Rather than feeling frustrated that I had to take more time off from work than planned, travel 45 minutes to the hospital and 45 minutes back (which, in the later weeks of my pregnancy wasn't always easy!) I decided to see it as a blessing. After all, I got to see my babies every couple of weeks and it was reassuring.

I know it's easier said than done, but try not to worry too much about all the things that might go wrong – you might find yourself down a Google rabbit hole of doom and end up feeling anxious, which won't help you or your babies. However, it's good to be prepared, and for some mums, knowing what could happen during their pregnancy helps to relieve their anxiety. Saying that, the 'big' complication that most pregnant twin mums are worried about developing is **Twin to Twin Transfusion Syndrome** (TTTS).

<u>TTTS</u>: The Facts

✸ TTTS affects 10 to 15 per cent of monochorionic twins (identical twins sharing a placenta).

✸ Non-identical twins, or identical twins with their own placentas, are not at risk.

✸ TTTS occurs when the blood vessels on the shared placenta supply each twin with an uneven amount of blood. Part of the blood flow is 'diverted' from one (donor) twin to the other (recipient) twin.

✸ TTTS can be dangerous for both twins – the lack of blood supply can affect the donor twin's growth and the recipient twin's heart can be put under strain.

✸ The treatment for early stage TTTS is often amnioreduction – when a fine needle drains excess amniotic fluid from the recipient twin.

✸ For more advanced stages, the treatment is laser ablation therapy, which involves closing off the blood vessels connecting the twins using a laser.

✸ Many TTTS pregnancies result in both twins being born full-term and healthy but there is a substantial risk to both twins. There are symptoms to look out for: your bump suddenly feeling bigger (overnight or in a day), feeling tight or looking shiny, and feeling breathless or having heart palpitations.

'I was diagnosed with Twin to Twin Transfusion Syndrome'

HANNAH, MUM TO FOUR-YEAR-OLD IDENTICAL TWINS

I was being scanned every two weeks during my pregnancy, and when I was 20 weeks pregnant, a scan showed that I had TTTS. I had to go straight to the specialist unit at a nearby hospital for more scans. On the way to the hospital I couldn't stop crying. I thought I was going to lose the babies. Within half an hour of getting there I was in the operating theatre, with lots of people in the room, getting ready to have laser ablation surgery. My husband was there, holding my hand, and it was explained to us that one, or both, of the babies might not survive. The procedure was done under local anaesthetic and during it I could see on the screen what they were doing but all I could feel were 'pops' in my belly. The consultant was so good at chatting to me and taking my mind off what was happening. Afterwards they checked the babies' heartbeats and told us that we wouldn't know whether the procedure had been a success until my next scan, a week later.

That week seemed to stretch out forever – I remember being up in the night and rubbing my tummy, thinking, 'I hope you're both OK!' I felt so nervous going for the scan a week later, and as soon as I was told both babies were fine and the surgery had worked I felt such relief. The rest of my pregnancy went much more smoothly, thankfully. I carried on having scans every two weeks but nothing abnormal showed on them and I delivered my twin girls by Caesarean section at 36 weeks.

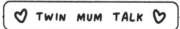

'My advice for you, if you're diagnosed with TTTS'

ANDIE, MUM OF IDENTICAL 22-MONTH-OLD TWIN GIRLS

Have hope. *We were lucky that our twin girls survived TTTS and have had no health issues. However some parents aren't so lucky and it is devastating. When we found out that we had Stage 3 TTTS at 20 weeks pregnant I named both of the babies. I spoke and sang to them constantly. Talking to them really helped me visualise our future with them, no matter the outcome, my girls were with me in those difficult times.*

Speak to other TTTS mums. *I got in touch with Twins Trust as soon as we found out we had TTTS and they put me in touch with someone who had been through the same experience. She'd been through TTTS and her babies had arrived safely. It helped to have someone to chat to who understood.*

Don't read all the negative stories! *It'll only stress you out and upset you even more. It's natural to want to turn to Google but it can be overwhelming and scary. We decided to focus on us, and not read too much into other stories and that helped a lot.*

Rest after laser ablation surgery. *My consultant advised a few days rest after the laser ablation, but in the USA they advise complete bed rest for as long as possible, so I decided to put myself on bed rest for two to three weeks and after that, I took things very easy – with baths, meditation and trying to relax.*

6 THINGS you could start thinking about now

1 **Ask your midwife if it's possible to get as many dates as possible for antenatal appointments now** - some hospitals are able to give you them right up until your due date.

2 **What kind of birth appeals to you**, and what conversations will you need to have at antenatal appointments about this?

3 **Think about logistics** - if you have a child or children, will you take them to appointments or arrange for someone to look after them?

4 **Speak to your employer** about getting time off for the appointments if you need to.

5 **Ask your midwife if they offer hand expressing/ colostrum harvesting packs** and how you get one - harvesting colostrum can be a great thing to do in the latter stages of a twin pregnancy.

6 **What does your 'fourth trimester' look like** (the first three months post-birth)? Think about what kind of support you'll have, and from who. Is there anything you need to put in place now, or are there conversations you can have with family members or friends who may be able to offer support?

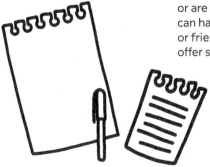

IF YOU ONLY DO 3 THINGS

1 Use your antenatal appointments well – plan what you want to ask and take your time when you're in there.

2 Listen to your body and rest when you need to.

3 Tune into your mental health and let your partner and family know how they can support you (see the next chapter for more on this).

Chapter 4

Looking after your mental health during pregnancy

One of the hardest things, for me, about the first trimester was this incredibly flat feeling I had. I didn't feel depressed at the time but I did feel like life was a bit . . . grey. Looking back, with hindsight, it was possibly mild antenatal depression I was experiencing.

Despite being over the moon that I was pregnant – especially considering it had taken five years of fertility treatment – I found it hard to feel excited about anything. Even being pregnant. I'd meet people in the street who'd congratulate me on my pregnancy, and chat about how excited I must be. 'Yes! So excited!' I'd fib. And as I walked away from the conversation, I'd be thinking: 'Hmm, I know I should be excited, but right now, I just feel tired and sick and a bit . . . meh about life.'

It felt like too much of a mental stretch to find joy in things. Instead, I found myself focusing on how nauseous I was feeling, how tired I was and how I'd gone off the taste of tea and chocolate (two of my favourite things in this world). I also had an internal Countdown-style clock ticking away, because I was so

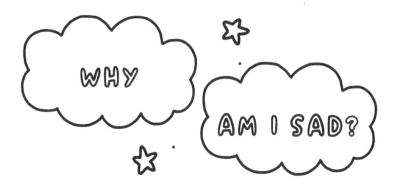

WHY AM I SAD?

desperate to get to the 12-week mark in the hope that I'd start to feel better around then and could start to enjoy my pregnancy.

When I was eight weeks pregnant we went on a little family break to the Peak District. It was the Easter holidays and we were hoping for a few days of glorious spring sunshine in the countryside. Instead, it was 24/7 fog, cold and I spent a lot of the week reading (and throwing up) while my husband entertained our daughter in the nearby swimming pool and soft play centre. Looking back, the holiday seemed to perfectly mirror my mood. A week that should have been beautiful, warm and filled with happy moments was foggy, cold and disappointing.

But something that brought a reassuring feeling of relief was that this was all familiar to me – I'd experienced the same thing when I'd been pregnant with my eldest. And back then it had lifted at around the Week 14 of pregnancy. When this happened, I remember describing it to friends as feeling like blinkers had been removed from my eyes. It was as if I'd been seeing the world in black and white for weeks, but suddenly I was seeing everything in colour again.

So I knew that it wasn't something that I should be particularly worried about, and thankfully, the same thing happened again

– the flat feeling started to fade away by the second trimester. In fact, around the same time that we were told we were having TWINS. As if mother nature was just enjoying this emotional roller coaster I was on. 'Sure, the grey flat feeling is fading now, but can I just throw in something else to really spice up your pregnancy?'

Even though this dip in mental health during my pregnancy was brief and mild, it gave me a small insight into what antenatal depression or anxiety must be like. Postnatal depression (see page 190 for more on this) is talked about a lot – and rightly so – but we don't hear about antenatal mental health quite so much. Yet it's a time of massive change. We have hormonal shifts happening, we're processing all of the information being given to us at appointments, we're thinking about how our lives are going to change, we're dealing with how we're physically feeling . . . it's not surprising so many of us feel emotionally wobbly during a pregnancy.

Twelve per cent of pregnant women suffer from some kind of antenatal depression or anxiety and many of those women are pregnant with twins – thanks to the extra worries about pregnancy complications, the financial implications and worrying about raising twins. In fact, research by Twins Trust shows that parents dealing with complications during pregnancy are twice as likely to suffer from mental health issues. Your midwife or GP may develop a mental health care plan and there may be extra support, like groups or therapy sessions, available to you during your pregnancy. Ask what there is in your area.

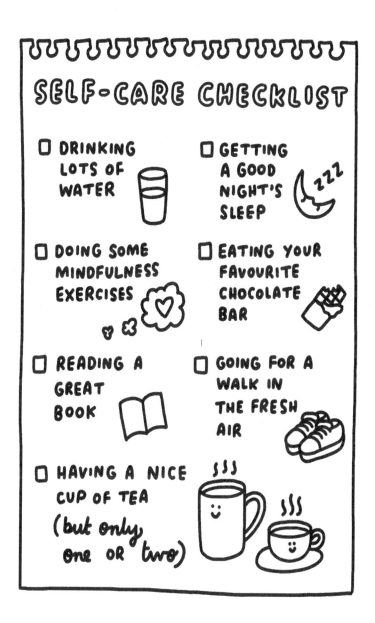

SELF-CARE CHECKLIST

- ☐ DRINKING LOTS OF WATER
- ☐ GETTING A GOOD NIGHT'S SLEEP
- ☐ DOING SOME MINDFULNESS EXERCISES
- ☐ EATING YOUR FAVOURITE CHOCOLATE BAR
- ☐ READING A GREAT BOOK
- ☐ GOING FOR A WALK IN THE FRESH AIR
- ☐ HAVING A NICE CUP OF TEA (but only one or two)

How I looked after *my* mental health during my twin pregnancy

❋ I made a big effort to 'tune into' my mental health – something many of us are, thankfully, better at doing these days. I asked myself how I was feeling every day and I tried to acknowledge my feelings, even if they seemed silly, confusing or insignificant.

❋ I lowered my expectations of how much I could do – both physically and mentally. If you're anything like me, you'll be used to buzzing about, seeing people, running errands, getting stuff done. When I was pregnant, my energy levels and mental state meant that I just wasn't up to doing much. But rather than beat myself up about it, I just accepted that life would be quieter for me until I felt a bit more like my normal self.

❋ I told my husband how I was feeling. I'm terrible at bottling up feelings and worries, but I chatted to my husband about this flat feeling I was experiencing, and even just the act of saying it out loud made me feel better. Having other people aware of your mental and emotional state is so important as they can look out for any dips and offer support.

❋ I went for regular walks – even if I wasn't feeling up to it, I would just do a short walk. The fresh air and endorphins made a huge difference to how I was feeling.

❋ I went to some 'Mindful Mums' workshops for expectant twin and multiple mums in my local town. Run by mental health charity MIND it was a great place to meet other twin mums and chat about what life as a twin mum would be like.

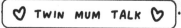

'I found my first trimester overwhelming and impossible'

SHAKIRA, MUM OF TWO AND PREGNANT WITH TWINS

I spent eight weeks of my first trimester in bed – partly because I had such bad nausea but it was also a mental health issue too. I have a phobia of being sick – so many people can feel nausea and just carry on with their day, but I'm not like that. I find it a very lonely and isolated place.

At six weeks I spoke to my midwife about how low and sick I was feeling and she said to get back in touch at nine weeks if I was still feeling bad. I spent the next three weeks just crying because I felt so sick. It was physically, emotionally and psychologically draining. It's totally overwhelming.

With mental health, it can just take one trigger – for me it was the nausea – and it can affect how you see everything. Everything felt impossible and I felt so alone. I have a great support network around me, and my family and husband tried to encourage me to get up and get on with looking after my two sons, but I literally couldn't. I was broken. I've got a history of OCD and one of my proudest achievements with this pregnancy is that it hasn't spiralled into kick-starting my OCD again. It's all down to breathing exercises and learning how to stay calm, no matter what is going on around me. I'm starting to feel a lot better now and I've asked my midwife for some extra mental-health support during the pregnancy. I'm also planning to book some hypnotherapy too. I'm determined to look after my mental health as much as I can during my twin pregnancy.

4 THINGS to remember about your mental health during your twin pregnancy

Dr Emma Svanberg (@mumologist), clinical psychologist

1 Don't underestimate how vulnerable a twin pregnancy can leave you. You're going through a monumental transition in life and you may be worried about additional stressors like disrupted sleep, financial pressures and the worry of looking after two babies.

2 If you have experienced a mental-health problem in the past, you are feeling unsupported, worried about your living situation or you have complications during your pregnancy, those things can all make you more likely to suffer from anxiety or low mood (and less commonly, obsessive compulsive disorders, or more acute difficulties such as bipolar disorder and psychosis).

3 If you are worried about your mental health, speak to your midwife about it and get the support you need. There may be specialist local mental-health services that can support you.

4 If you have supportive relationships with your partner, family and friends, let them know how they can help you. If you find it hard to think about what could feel supportive (it's often hard to know what can help), sometimes just having space to talk about how you're feeling and have someone validate and listen can be powerful.

I'M **WORRIED** ABOUT...

WHO I CAN *talk* TO ABOUT THIS...

ONE THING I CAN DO TO *feel better* ABOUT THIS IS...

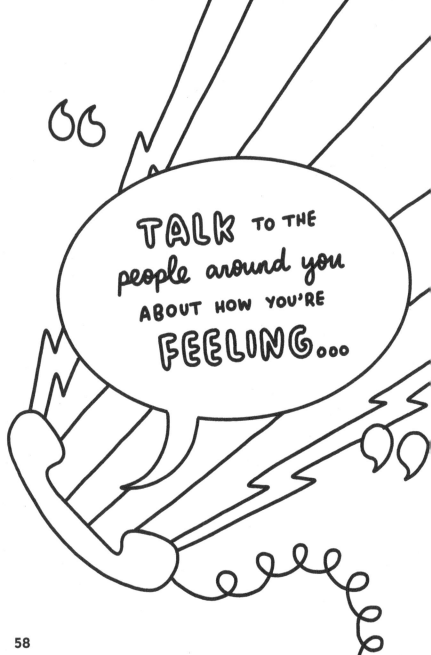

IF YOU ONLY DO 3 THINGS

1 Talk to the people around you about how you're feeling.

2 If you're worried and feel you need extra support, speak to your midwife.

3 Check out what's available locally in the way of classes and therapy.

Chapter 5

Eating for three?

I'm sure we've all heard the phrase, 'Eating for two' – when a pregnant mum ups her calorie intake because she is growing a human. So when we're pregnant with two humans, that means HAPPY DAYS! We can eat loads more, right?

Well . . . sadly not. And actually, if you're anything like me, you probably won't even feel like eating lots. During my first twin trimester all I could stomach was bland, carby food. I ate bowl after bowl of Coco Pops (and focused on all that calcium I was getting from the milk!) along with toast, jacket potatoes and what felt like endless packets of ready-salted Hula Hoops and Mini Cheddars. My taste buds changed and things that I usually love, like cups of tea and bars of chocolate, suddenly left me feeling disinterested.

I felt worried that I wasn't eating as much fruit and veg as I should have been. I mean, I'm the kind of person who feels guilty when I don't manage my five a day, but add to that the extra mum-guilt of, 'My unhealthy diet might be damaging my unborn babies,' and it was major. But chatting to a midwife friend reminded me that I shouldn't be so worried. 'The first trimester is a bit like one long hangover,' she told me. 'It's normal to struggle to eat healthy foods, but try not to worry. You'll feel better in your second trimester and you can make up for it then and eat a nice variety of healthy foods.' Phew!

And she was right. As I moved into my second trimester my taste buds reverted back to normal, and I was able to eat a much bigger variety of flavours and foods. I celebrated by getting my husband to take me out for lunch! 'Let's go to that nice café by the station,' I told him. 'I want a proper lunch!' I ordered avocado on toast with chilli and feta (and then spent half an hour googling: 'Can you eat feta cheese when pregnant?' and not getting a definitive answer so I left the feta on the side of the plate, just in case). It felt good to be out and about eating a normal lunch in a normal cafe again.

As my pregnancy progressed, one thing I wasn't expecting, was being unable to eat large meals (I'm used to having a very healthy appetite!) and I was much happier grazing on small meals throughout the day.

Eating for two is a myth!

Official guidelines on both singleton and twin pregnancies are that energy needs don't change in the first six months of pregnancy and that women only require around 200 extra calories per day in the last trimester of pregnancy (which is the equivalent to two pieces of wholegrain toast with olive oil spread or a small handful of nuts, seeds and dried fruit). Which means that the whole 'eating for two' thing is a total myth!

It's also advised that pregnant women drink at least two litres of water every day, and pregnant twin mums are advised to drink a couple of glasses more than this. It's such a good idea to carry around a refillable water bottle whenever you go out. When it comes to supplements, pregnant women are advised to take folic acid until the twelfth week of the pregnancy to help prevent birth defects, and it's no different for twin mums. You should be able to get all the vitamins and nutrients you need from your diet but if you're concerned you can take a supplement like Pregnacare.

What you <u>need to know</u> about nutrition during your twin pregnancy

Charlotte Stirling-Reed (@sr_nutrition), registered nutritionist and expert in maternal and child nutrition

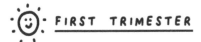 **FIRST TRIMESTER**

Try not to put too much pressure or guilt on yourself if you're feeling too nauseous to eat well – that won't help anyone

A lot of the nutrients that your babies will need will come from your body's stores – stores that were created prior to you becoming pregnant.

Do what you can to look after yourself, rest and get fluids in. Looking after your health and listening to your body is important too. If you can, try eating little and often and sipping on fluids slowly, throughout the day.

Boost plain food with nutrients if you can

Dry and plain foods can really help some pregnant women as they are often less triggering of the nausea, but do what you can to boost the nutrients you're having alongside them. For example, if dry crackers or toast are your thing, can you top it with cheese or peanut butter to add a few extra nutrients? You can also try herbal teas, which some women swear by for pregnancy nausea – peppermint, ginger and chamomile are all refreshing options. When it comes to herbal teas, try to vary them and opt for no more than four herbal teas a day.

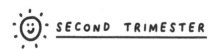 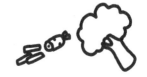

SECOND TRIMESTER

It's all about finding a balance
There's no magic diet needed during pregnancy, just simple healthy eating. Balancing out the food groups and staying hydrated as much as possible. Variety is always key and can really help you get the vitamins, minerals and energy and proteins you need to grow your healthy babies. Try smoothie bowls with nuts and seeds, salads packed with veggies and soups and stews.

Keep your energy levels up
Energy is so important during pregnancy – especially with twins! Try to eat regularly and try not to skip meals (where possible!) as this is the best way to make sure you can top up your energy levels. Carbohydrates are a fab source of energy, try to opt for wholegrains such as brown rice, wholemeal pasta or oats.

Eat iron-rich foods
Make sure you get your iron levels checked with your GP or midwife – if you were low in iron before you become pregnant, or haven't been eating enough iron-rich foods you might need a supplement. In terms of dietary sources, meat, especially red meat, is a good source. Additionally, foods such as lentils, beans and chickpeas are a good source of iron and are great options if you're plant-based. Porridge oats and fortified cereals are also good options as a source of iron.

Eat five a day to stay regular!
Constipation is a regular complaint during pregnancy, especially around the second trimester, but it can occur at anytime. If it's affecting you a lot, make sure you see your GP. Drinking plenty of fluids and also eating lots of fruits and vegetables can really make a difference. It sounds like dull advice, but getting your five a day each day can really help to make you more regular. Wholegrains such as oats, nuts, seeds, lentils and beans may also help as they contain plenty of fibre.

63

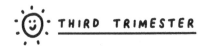 **THIRD TRIMESTER**

Have smaller meals if you need to

Try to avoid grazing throughout the day and try to stick to regular mealtimes, mainly because this can help you to keep track of what you're eating and you'll know if you've included all the food groups (e.g. carbs, proteins, fruit and veggies) that you need. Stick with those regular times to eat, or simply add a few extra occasions for snacks into your day. Focus on nutrient-rich options where possible to help with pregnancy symptoms and also with topping up your intakes.

5 super-quick nutrient-rich snack ideas for when you're at home	5 easy nutrient-rich snack ideas to take out and about
• A banana and a dollop of peanut butter • Plain yogurt topped with berries • Baked beans on toast • Slice of toasted fruit bread or malt loaf • Wholemeal pitta bread with hummus	• A mini bag of nuts and raisins • Oatcakes and an apple • Dried apricots • Sticks of celery, carrot, red pepper and cucumber • Make a smoothie to go – blend a pot of plain yogurt with a small banana, a peeled nectarine, peeled kiwi and some raspberries. Add a splash of milk.

Dear ....

·THESE· ARE THE FOODS AND DRINKS I'M _really_ MISSING RIGHT NOW. SO ONCE THE BABIES ARE HERE, THIS IS A LITTLE REQUEST FOR THE FOLLOWING MEAL:

AND A NICE GLASS OF:

THANK YOU _so much!_
I CAN ALMOST TASTE IT NOW, JUST THINKING ABOUT IT.

Love from .... ✗

FOODS TO AVOID

There are certain foods that it's advised to avoid when pregnant (but don't worry - you'll soon be gorging on soft cheese again!).

Unpasteurised dairy products may contain a bacteria called listeria which can cause an infection that is dangerous to unborn babies. Avoid foods like Brie, Camembert and chevre (unless cooked), soft blue cheeses (unless cooked), any unpasteurised cow's milk, goats' milk or sheep's milk or food made from it like soft goat's cheese.

Raw or undercooked meat, liver, all kinds of pâté (even veggie pâté), game meat - undercooked meat carries a risk of you getting toxoplasmosis which can lead to miscarriage. Liver has vitamin A which is dangerous to an unborn child and game meat might contain shot.

Uncooked or partially cooked (soft) eggs that don't have a British Lion Stamp on them. Eggs with the stamp can be eaten soft-cooked, as they're less likely to give you salmonella. You should avoid soft-cooked duck, goose or quail eggs.

Eat no more than two portions of oily fish a week (e.g. salmon, trout, mackerel and herring) - they can have pollutants, dioxins and polychlorinated biphenyls in them. Eat no more than two tuna steaks or four medium-size cans of tuna a week - it has more mercury in it than other fish.

Avoid certain fish and seafood altogether. Raw shellfish can have harmful bacteria, viruses or toxins in them. Shark, swordfish and marlin should also be avoided because they have high levels of mercury.

Limit caffeine to no more than 200mg per day, which is roughly two mugs of instant coffee or two and a half mugs of tea.

IF YOU ONLY DO 3 THINGS

1. Don't feel guilty about what you're able to (or not able to) eat in the first trimester.

2. Keep your energy levels up with healthy snacks.

3. Stay regular with lots of fibre from fruit and veg!

Chapter 6

Looking after your growing bump

Watching your body changing during pregnancy can be such a tricky time for lots of us – we've grown up surrounded by messages from the media and advertising telling us that slim is beautiful and many of us have struggled over the years trying to reach that (not always attainable) goal. Back in the day, I'd have loved to have had a tummy flat enough to wear crop tops like Paris Hilton and I tried so hard to have thighs and bum small enough to wear miniskirts like Cheryl Tweedy, but I eventually realised that dieting and guilting myself into exercise was making me miserable.

So when I was pregnant for the first time and I found myself feeling good about my belly getting bigger it was such a weird experience. I wasn't used to celebrating my body expanding in size, having been conditioned for so long to think that small = good.

With my twin pregnancy my bump started showing much sooner – but I still had the weird 'inbetweeny' stage at around 13 to 14 weeks when my bump had started to grow but it wasn't quite big enough to look like a proper bump. Lots of my regular clothes no longer fitted but maternity clothes were enormous on me. I found myself patting and holding my stomach a lot, as if to emphasise the tiny bump, and to make myself 'look pregnant', when actually I just looked a bit rounder than usual. It triggered all sorts of deep-rooted issues for me: 'What if people think I've just put on weight?' I'd worry as I got dressed and looked in my full-length mirror from various angles. Which is clearly bonkers, because a) putting on weight isn't something to be ashamed of, and b) I was growing two humans inside there, which frankly is something to be celebrated.

And I think that's the key thing here. If you're looking in the mirror, like I did, and you're feeling a bit rubbish about your body shape changing, try to think about the amazing thing that your body is doing right now. It's growing

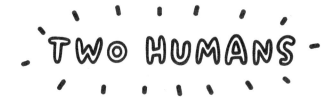

TWO! Not even one! Growing one human is incredible enough as it is, but two?! Think about the mind-blowing series of events that have led up to this moment. Whether it happened inside your body or with help from fertility doctors, an egg has been fertilised and then split into two, or two eggs have been fertilised, and they've attached themselves firmly in the lining of your womb, where the cells have multiplied and developed into embryos. Now, they're growing into two babies. Isn't that mad?!

So when you look in the mirror, try to look past any body-image issues you might have and think about how amazing your body is. Did you know that a 2015 study by the University of Michigan found that giving birth to a baby (just the one) is as hard on the body as running a marathon? And while we don't all have vaginal deliveries, for lots of twin mums it's an option, which means giving birth to twins is even harder on the body than running a marathon. Us. Twin. Mums. Are. Rock. Stars. (I had a Caesarean section with my twins but I'm going to bask in the twin mum glory here regardless!)

And speaking of exercise, something else that might make you feel better about your twin pregnancy body is getting it moving. Of course, you could be reading this and feeling exhausted, nauseous and you could be thinking that getting moving is the last thing you're able to do right now. But exercise doesn't have to mean a punishing gym session or a body combat class.

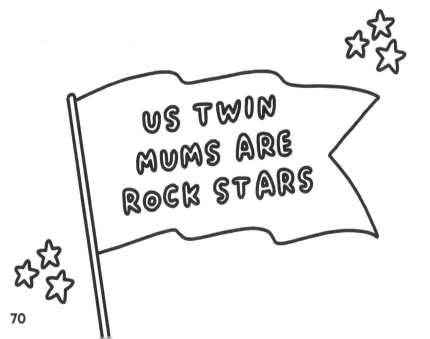

<u>WHY</u> & <u>HOW</u> to exercise during your twin pregnancy

Ante- and postnatal fitness expert Shakira Akabusi (@shakira.akabusi) shares her tips and experience

I'm currently 14 weeks pregnant with twins and believe me when I say that I haven't felt like moving my body at all during the past few weeks. I'm just too tired. It's been enough just getting up, getting my kids dressed, getting them to school, coming home and cleaning the house. By the time I've done that it's 12pm and I need to sit down for an hour.

My body is exhausted.

It's important to listen to your body and just have a real respect for the fact that it's going through a lot. Twin pregnancy is a workout in itself. Your body is creating something incredible and that is taking so much energy. So have respect for the process and be willing to take a break.

But, when you are feeling up to it, there are so many benefits to exercising during your twin pregnancy. In terms of immediate effects, it can give you a mood boost and an energy boost – so don't see it as 'I'm too tired to exercise,' see it as 'I'm tired so I'll exercise to boost my energy.' Even simply sitting outdoors, and feeling sunshine on your face can help to boost feelings of positivity and health. Fresh air has been proven to boost a person's mood, strengthen the immune system, aid digestion and increase energy levels.

If you feel you can, get your limbs moving and go for a walk. Even just five or ten minutes. I took my dog for a ten-minute walk the other day, and when I came back I was exhausted. So take it gently.

For some people walking is enough but others might feel up to doing more. It's important to do low-impact exercise like yoga or swimming and avoid traditional abdominal exercises like sit-ups and crunches. It's a good idea, though, to exercise the abdominal muscles in a certain way during pregnancy as it helps to control the tilt of the pelvis, stabilise the spine and support the pregnant uterus, as well as helping to reduce backache due to the increased lumbar curvature.

Exercises like pelvic tilts, four-point kneeling with single arm lifts, side-lying hip hitch and adapted half plank are good, safe abdominal exercises when pregnant. Working on your core muscles can help with diastasis recti (the gap between the abdominal muscles that many women have in the postnatal period).

As you probably already know, pregnancy stimulates lots of hormonal changes for women, and one of these hormones is relaxin. Production of relaxin starts at around the second week of pregnancy and its role is to relax the ligaments of the pelvic floor in preparation for childbirth. But because relaxin cannot confine its effects to just the pelvic area, it means that joint stability throughout your entire body is affected.

So it's important to take care to control the range of movement when exercising – the stability of your once-solid joint structures has been compromised.

If you're worried about putting on weight in pregnancy try to understand that it's a temporary change, your body is doing something amazing and postnatally there is so much you can do to create a body that you are proud of and that you are comfortable with.

YOUR PREGNANCY MANTRAS

I AM A **STRONG,** *healthy,* WOMAN.

MY **BODY** WAS *designed* TO **NOURISH,** *protect,* AND GROW MY BABIES.

I LOVE MY PREGNANT BODY - IT'S *beautiful* + IT'S EQUIPPED WITH *everything* I NEED TO TAKE CARE OF MY BABIES.

I AM **PROUD** OF *myself* FOR BEING ABLE TO *carry,* *nurture,* & *sustain* A LIFE WITHIN ME.

I *allow myself* TO SEE THE **BEAUTY** + **JOY** IN THIS PROCESS.

WRITE YOUR OWN BODY MANTRAS AND STICK THEM ON YOUR MIRROR.

How to do a gentle Pilates squat

Lots of pregnant mums discover that yoga and Pilates are brilliant for getting them moving and stretching in a gentle way, and for easing pregnancy aches and pains. Anya Hayes (@mothers.wellness.toolkit), Pilates instructor and mum of two, loves this squat for gaining the strength you'll need in later pregnancy – and if you're giving birth vaginally.

'The Pilates squat is possibly the most important birthing exercise you can do. It helps to open your pelvis, strengthens your thighs, hips and knees and challenges your stamina. Make sure you don't overdo it, *but do challenge your endurance as much as you can*, breathing softly and deeply through any discomfort.'

1. Stand correctly, arms relaxed by your sides, palms facing in towards your thighs.

2. Breathe in to lengthen the spine. Bend the knees and hips simultaneously and hinge forwards from the hips. Lengthen the arms slightly forwards.

3. Breathe out and straighten through the backs of the legs to stand upright once more.

4. Repeat up to 10 times.

Be careful of squatting too deeply if your babies are low in the pelvis or if you have any symptoms of pelvic organ prolapse, and don't ever ignore pelvic pain. Listen to your body and stay high if you feel any discomfort: make sure your back remains lengthened and hinge into the hip joints as if you're sitting down in a chair.

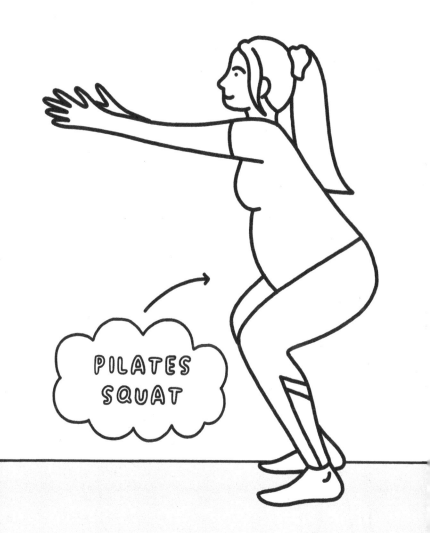

PILATES
SQUAT

How to dress your twin bump

Even if you've always been really relaxed and happy about your body, pregnancy can throw up issues. Not least . . .

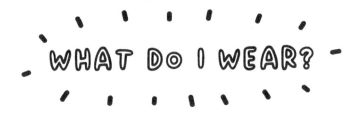

Perhaps you're one of the lucky ones who can make their pre-pregnancy wardrobe work for them? I was never that chic or inventive! I did, however, love being pregnant because it was the only time ever in my life that I've been able to wear tight, body-con dresses and fitted tops. But I still found clothing and outfits a bit of a challenge during pregnancy.

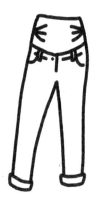

 FIRST TRIMESTER

I felt so green around the gills and exhausted, that I didn't care what I wore. My go-to outfit was jeans and a jumper. Any desire to look stylish went firmly out of the window. But on any day where I had to make an effort, I'd bung on some red lipstick (to distract from my grey pallor) and wear my trusty stretchy pleather leggings, sweatshirt and comfy trainers.

☀ SECOND TRIMESTER

As my bump started to expand and my normal jeans and dresses no longer fitted, I started to buy some maternity clothing. But – unless you're rolling in cash – you can't just buy a whole new wardrobe, can you? So I spent the next few months rotating the same few outfits – and it's totally OK to do this. Don't feel you have to create an extensive maternity wardrobe. A few basics jazzed up with some accessories can go a long way! It's such a shame, though, that shopping for maternity clothes is not always fun. You're suddenly limited to teeny-tiny sections of shops, with only a few things to choose from, and what are the chances that those things are clothes you like and that suit you? When you think about how many women are pregnant on any given day (there were over half a million pregnancies in 2018 in just England and Wales) you'd think retailers would be able to offer a bigger and more varied range of maternity clothing.

☀ THIRD TRIMESTER

Like many twin mums, my third trimester wasn't actually a whole trimester – it was eight weeks, and at least six of those were spent not moving much from the sofa! So I spent a lot of time in stretchy cotton maternity jumpsuits and maternity jogging bottoms.

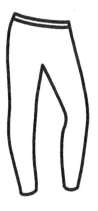

Which is ironic considering most of that sofa-time was spent watching *Suits* and lusting after the sharp workwear outfits worn by Meghan Markle and co.

KEY PIECES for every twin pregnancy maternity wardrobe

Charlotte Kewley (@charlottekewley), fashion stylist and mum of two

It's not worth investing in a whole new wardrobe that will last for around six months. But with twins, you know from the off that you're most likely not going to have a tiny petite bump, so invest from the beginning to ensure you get the most wear (and the most comfort). The key pieces that I think are worth getting are:

BLACK LEGGINGS

A pair of over-the-bump leggings that offer support and look flattering. They'll grow with you. Perfect for dress-down days but also easy to 'style up'. I'm a big fan of leggings with a good-length top/shirt and then a smarter more tailored coat over the top to make them look less like loungewear. Worth buying a good quality pair if you can as they'll wash well and last your entire pregnancy and beyond.

JEANS

I think most women want a good pair of maternity jeans to see them through. Ideally two pairs – under-the-bump for the first half of the pregnancy and then over-the-bump as you want a little more support and coverage. You can get maternity versions of every jeans style, so choose whichever are your preference. You can spend lots on these but actually I think you can get some really good maternity jeans without breaking the bank.

A JUMPSUIT OR DUNGAREES

I appreciate these aren't for everyone but there's nothing more comfortable (with or without a bump) than a soft jumpsuit or dungarees. And there are so many excellent ones now, both on the

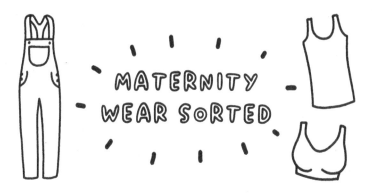

MATERNITY WEAR SORTED

high street and from independent maternity brands. Just type 'jersey maternity jumpsuit' into Google and you can thank me later.

MATERNITY BRAS

Soft, comfortable and they can be underwired or not, depending on your preference. A must. The high street do some great ones and you don't need to spend a lot.

LONG MATERNITY VESTS

These are the secret weapon of many a pregnant mum! You can layer these under any top or jumper and it means you can continue to wear regular tops for longer without constantly flashing your bump. With twin pregnancies it means you might be able to get away with wearing normal tops until your 20-week point, or beyond, depending on your bump size.

MATERNITY TIGHTS

To wear with dresses.

DRESSES

But this doesn't have to be a maternity dress. If your style is wearing more bohemian/floaty dresses they may continue to work for most of your pregnancy. If you prefer a more structured dress it can be good to invest in one or two.

Charlotte's Top Tips

❋ **It's good to have maybe three favourite looks** – a jeans look, a leggings look and a smarter look – and then buy a few things to be able to mix them up, like a couple of T-shirt options that work and chuck-on accessories to make them feel different.

❋ **Use accessories to make yourself feel like 'you'.** Some bright lipstick, eyeliner flicks, jewellery or a hat always help to make a maternity look feel like your style.

❋ **The pre-loved and rental fashion market is growing by the day**, and there are so many great maternity options in good condition because they haven't been worn much. Consider renting for parties or events (rather than wearing a pricey maternity dress once) and look at buying pre-loved for the rest of your maternity wardrobe too. It'll work out cheaper and you'll be helping the environment.

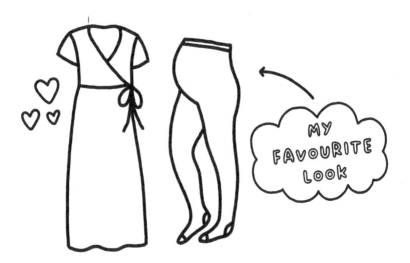

MY FAVOURITE LOOK

DRAW YOU WITH YOUR TWIN BUMP
WEARING YOUR FAVOURITE OUTFIT:

LoVE YouR BuMP

Try to take five minutes every day to appreciate what your body is doing right now. This mini-exercise is quick and when done daily will make a huge difference to your twin pregnancy confidence levels.

* When you're getting dressed stand in front of a mirror (full-length, if possible) in your undies.

* Rub body oil or your favourite body moisturiser, in a clockwise motion, into your bump and the surrounding areas – your hips, round to your back.

* As you're doing this, say one thing you love about your body out loud, and thank your body for growing your babies and looking after them until they're ready to be born.

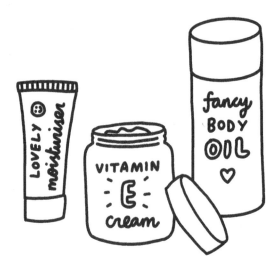

IF YOU ONLY DO 3 THINGS

1. Look in the mirror and tell yourself that your body is doing something incredible.

2. Get moving – go for a gentle walk or do some yoga or swimming.

3. Rummage in your accessories drawer and see if you can discover a long-forgotten scarf or necklace that you love.

Chapter 7

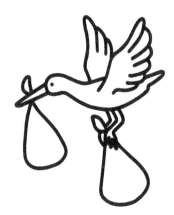

Planning for life with twins

Sitting on the sofa with my husband, cup of (decaf) tea in one hand, Jaffa Cake in the other, I wailed, '*But it's just so much to sort out!*'

I was around 17 weeks pregnant and we'd decided to sit down one evening to go through what we needed to organise and buy ahead of the twins arriving. Which was great in theory, but in reality it meant that all of those things that I'd been carefully sweeping under the fluffy carpet of my brain suddenly had nowhere to hide. Tears streamed down my face – I felt totally overwhelmed and the sheer enormity of everything that had to be done and organised seemed unmanageable.

'We have to research double buggies: do we want an in-line buggy or a side-by-side? Will a side-by-side buggy fit through our front door? We have to work out whether we can fit two infant car seats and a high-backed booster into our car, we need to research infant car seats, we might need to buy a new car! Do we need one Moses basket or will they sleep in the same one?' I was speaking at around 300mph. 'Do we need two of everything?!' I asked him. (The answer to that, by the way is no! There are some things you might want two of – we had two Moses baskets, two slings, two bouncer chairs – but other things like playmats and toys, we bought one of (see page 88).

'Well, first,' my husband said gently, 'just breathe. Stop and breathe.'

He made me another cup of tea and we made a plan. I'd research buggies. He'd research car seats. I'd look around at cots. He'd start clearing out and redecorating the room that would become the twins' bedroom. We wrote a list of everything we'd need to buy, and I noted down what we had one of already. Just getting it all down on paper, in black and white, and making a plan made it seem less daunting.

In my head, I'd been focused on **EVERYTHING** that needed to be done. But in reality I didn't have to do everything by myself and I didn't have to do everything right now. Once we divided up tasks and worked out what could be done now and what could wait the task seemed much more manageable.

It can be so overwhelming when you think about all the preparation and planning you need to put in place before the arrival of your twins. Even if you've already done it once before (like we had!) the logistics of having two small babies on their way can throw your once-confident mind into a panic.

If you haven't already heard of Twins Trust (formerly known as TAMBA), then now is the time to look them up. They're an invaluable source of support and advice for twin mums and dads, with online and in-person courses on everything from preparing for parenthood, breastfeeding, sleep and more (look them up at **twinstrust.org**).

Here's Louise Bowman from Twins Trust sharing her tips on planning for twins . . .

How to navigate planning for twins, <u>stress-free</u>!

Louise Bowman, Family Support Senior Coordinator, Twins Trust

YOU DON'T HAVE TO BUY EVERYTHING NOW

The important things are car seats and the buggy, clothes, blankets and cots/Moses baskets so that the babies have somewhere to sleep. Also, you might want to start stocking up on nappies and wipes because you will go through a lot. Other things can wait!

GET PERSONAL RECOMMENDATIONS FROM OTHER TWIN PARENTS

One of the best ways to research which kit to buy is speaking to other parents of twins. Go onto your local twins club Facebook page and ask for recommendations. Or visit your local twins club in person. I actually stopped someone in a shopping centre when I was pregnant to ask about her buggy! Speaking to parents who have been through it helps when you're making a decision.

THINK ABOUT WHAT YOU NEED TO SUIT YOUR LIFE

With the buggy, are you out walking a lot? Do you want tandem or side by side? Are you getting on the bus a lot? Do you need something that will fit a buggy board? Will it fit into the boot of your car? What's right for one set of twin parents might not be perfect for you.

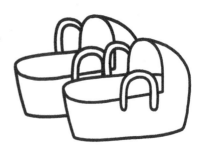

BUY SECONDHAND!

When we had our twins most of our equipment was secondhand. You have to buy new mattresses for all cots and Moses baskets and car seats also have to be bought new, unless you know for certain they have not been involved in an accident. We had my daughter's old car seat and then borrowed another from a trusted friend. So it's possible to get everything you need without spending a fortune. eBay and twin club sales are great places to look for a bargain.

YOU DON'T NEED TO BUY TWO OF EVERYTHING

With things like the Jumperoo, we bought one and we'd have one twin in it, while the other was on the play mat and then we'd swap them around.

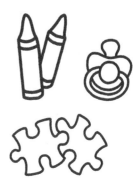

BOOK YOURSELF ONTO A COURSE!

Doing the Twins Trust Practical Preparing for Parenthood seminar or webinar is a great idea. They're available across the whole country, run by parents of twins and they're only two hours long. They're brilliant for preparing you for having two babies - looking at feeding, sleep, equipment needed and everything in between.

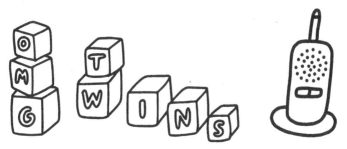

WHAT KIT DO I NEED?

It can be overwhelming when you start thinking about what you need to buy for one baby, let alone two! Which things do you need two of, and which do you only need one of? Here are the things that I couldn't have done without . . .

* **Double breast pump** (if you're planning to breastfeed/ express) to express more quickly

* **Twin feeding pillow** (great for breast- or bottle-feeding)

* **Steriliser for bottles** (I used a microwave one)

* **Bottles** for expressed milk or infant formula

* **Breast pads** (lots)

* **Muslins** (lots)

* **Nappies and wipes** (lots)

* **Nappy cream**

* **One changing mat** (you can only change one baby at a time after all) or a second one if you want to have one in the living room and one in the bedroom

* **Twin baby carrier** OR **two single carriers/slings** if you're likely to only babywear when there are two of you around

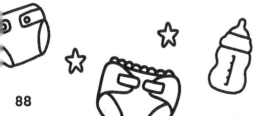

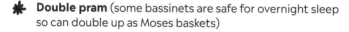

- **Two rear-facing infant car seats** (if you have a car)

- **Double pram** (some bassinets are safe for overnight sleep so can double up as Moses baskets)

- **Large changing bag** (we loved a rucksack version so it left both arms free!)

- **Large playmat** that both babies can play on at the same time

- **Two bouncy chairs** (so useful for soothing two babies at once – I used my feet to rock them!)

- **One baby bath** (you can buy a second later when they're too big to bathe together)

- **Two Moses baskets** (or one larger cot/travel cot if they're sharing to start with)

- **Dummies/soothers** if you use them (we had different designs for each baby)

- **One baby monitor**

Top tip from Karen, mum to eight-year-old identical twins
When you're having twins, don't buy a new pram. Buy a secondhand pram because over the course of the first few years you'll probably need two or three different prams and buggies. So don't think, 'That pram is going to be the pram that works for me for the whole two years or three years or four years.' Instead, buy one secondhand that'll work for the first year, sell it and buy another one. I remember buying an iCandy from eBay and then reselling it for almost the same amount!

COMMON CONCERNS

Of course, it's not just worries about what to buy that can flood your mind (usually at 3am when pregnancy insomnia kicks in). Other common twin pregnancy concerns include:

Common concern	My advice
Where will they sleep?	There's a whole chapter on sleep (page 202) but in a nutshell, you can have your twins in a Moses basket each, in your bedroom, to start with or (like we did) have them sharing a bigger cot to start with. Then, when they're too big for that, they can sleep in a cot each.
Will I ever sleep again?	**YES!** As I'm writing this, my twins are roughly 18 months old and I get a full nine hours every night. That's not a promise that you will – lots of babies (twin or not) have sleeping issues up until school age, but the good news is that having twins doesn't automatically mean zero sleep forever more.
What if they cry at the same time?	This will happen a lot (see page 212) and you'll get used to: a) cuddling two babies at once and b) sharing the soothing with your partner – or whoever happens to be around.

Common concern	My advice
Will they nap at the same time?	They might. They might not. I found having low expectations of napping during the day was the best way – I'd assume that they'd nap at different times and if they slept at the same time, it was a bonus. The plus side of naps at different times is lovely one-to-one time with each baby!
How do you feed two babies at once?	See pages 150–151 and page 156 for an explanation on how to breastfeed and bottle-feed twins! It can be done!
What if the doorbell goes when I'm feeding them?	Some mums stick a note on the door to say they're busy with their babies, others just ignore the doorbell.
How will I feed them while out and about?	I timed going out around feeds so that I could feed at home, simply to make things easier for myself, but I did feed my twins in a cafe a few times and found that feeding them one at a time was easier than trying to tandem breastfeed. Bottle-feeding twins when out is easier if you have another pair of hands to help out.

Common concern	My advice
How will I fit on the bus with a double pram?	If you get on buses a lot, consider an in-line pram rather than a side-by-side pram, but be ready to let a few buses go by, if they already have a pram/buggy onboard and don't have space for you.
What if I need to use public loos when I'm out?	I got really good at going for a wee before going out with my twins, and then holding it in until I got home (I know, terrible!) but some public loos have large accessible cubicles that you can fit a double pram in.
How do I get them both from car to indoors if I'm on my own?	Some twin mums flex their super muscles and carry two car seats at once. Others take one car seat, lock the car, do a quick dash indoors and then come back for the second car seat.
Will we manage to choose two names we like?	It's harder than you might think, right? So much to consider. See below for more on this!

Choosing names for your twins

Picking a name for one unborn baby is a big deal, but two?

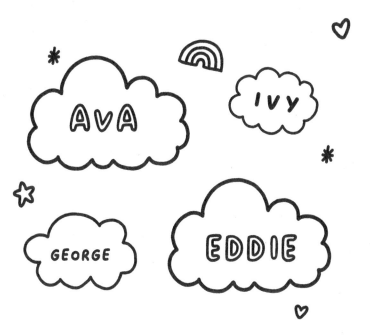

There's a lot to consider . . . do you make the names match in some way? Should they start with the same letter? Or rhyme? Perhaps they could be linked in some other way, e.g. a flower name or a biblical name for each twin. We opted for two totally unlinked names – but they do both start with a vowel, so in that sense, they kind of flow as you say them together.

The impact of the names you choose for your twins

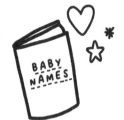

Dr Martha Deiros Collado, clinical psychologist (@dr.mdc_psychologist)

There haven't been many twin studies looking at the impact of names on their identity but when names are linked, it may reinforce the idea that they have a close union and this is likely to shape others expectations of them 'getting on well' with each other. This may make twin relationships tricky, particularly if they do not get on in adult life and/or have separate interests.

There's been some research done exploring the impact of names on how others perceive them and how they 'embody' their name through their actions and personality. However, most research in this area is flawed and limited because it's really difficult to disentangle nature from nurture.

What we do know is that the labels we use are socially constructed and infer meaning and expectations about who we are culturally and socio-economically and that they place gender expectations on us. For example, the name Rose and the name Alexandra may have different social expectations associated with them – Rose may lead to gender expectations of femininity, while Alexandra (often shortened to Alex) may feel more free to question gender stereotypes.

But ultimately all labels, including names, are socially constructed and this creates social expectations of who the person carrying the name is. With twins, having linked names may add an additional layer of expectation in terms of their relationship, which may be more or less useful depending on how their relationship develops and who they grow to be.

IF YOU ONLY DO 3 THINGS

1 Don't stress about organising everything now. You have time.

2 Check out local and online courses.

3 Look on eBay, Gumtree and local selling groups on Facebook for items you need.

PRE-BIRTH JOURNAL

I'M FEELING:

I'M WEARING:

I'M EATING:

I'M **EXCITED** ABOUT:

I'M nervous ABOUT:

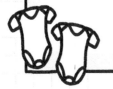

BIRTH

- - - - - - - -

It's nearly here. It's almost time to give birth to your twins. But before you do, read through this section to help you plan the kind of twin birth you want (even if your options appear limited), mentally prepare yourself and think about the hours and days that follow the birth. The aim of this part of the book is to inform and reassure you - knowledge is power, right?

Chapter 8

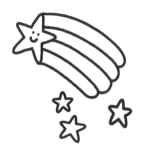

Planning your twin birth

Planning a birth can feel like such an abstract, weird concept. Planning a twin birth? Even more so! If you've never given birth before, then aside from watching episodes of *One Born Every Minute*, you'll probably have no idea what to expect, so how are you meant to know what kind of birth you want? And if you have given birth before, chances are, it was a singleton birth and giving birth to twins is a whole different kettle of fish, right? But . . .

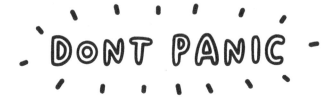

There are a few things that will determine the kind of birth that will be recommended to you and a few things for you to consider. In terms of timings, national guidelines state that if you're having monochorionic twins, elective birth (Caesarean or vaginal) should be offered at 36 weeks and if you're having dichorionic twins, elective birth should be offered at 37 weeks. It might be necessary to deliver the babies earlier if their health (or yours) is at risk.

During my twin pregnancy, I knew pretty much right from the off that the plan for my birth was a Caesarean section. At my 12-week scan, when they discovered I was having monochorionic twins, one of the first things that the consultant told me was that she recommended a C-section. Some people would have been disappointed – after all, lots of women really want to give birth vaginally. But I was relieved to be told the plan was a C-section. My eldest daughter had been born vaginally seven years earlier and I'd found the experience a lot harder than I'd expected to. On paper, it had been a bit of a textbook birth – nothing unusual happened – but it was a 31-hour labour, which left me feeling exhausted and shell-shocked.

Everyone is different though. You might be reading this and thinking you want your birth to be as natural as possible. You might feel that giving birth vaginally is something you want to experience.

You might have read about the benefits of a vaginal delivery: babies pick up good bacteria from the birth canal; excess fluid is squeezed from their lungs, which helps their digestive system and immune system; and mum has less healing to do so has a shorter stay in hospital.

You may feel like giving birth vaginally is how it's meant to be – it's what our body is designed for, after all! You might just have this gut instinct that a vaginal birth is what you want and you can't even articulate why.

But I was happy and relieved that giving birth this time would be different.

Midwife Q&A

With midwife and twin specialist Layla Toomer

Q DO I HAVE TO HAVE A CAESAREAN?

This is such a common question from twin mums and the answer is absolutely not. We would always encourage and support a vaginal birth. I think it's so important for mums to have the birth they want, so long as it's appropriate for them. It's important that you're fully informed about the risks and benefits of the Caesarean birth and the vaginal birth. There are lots of reasons that your doctor might recommend a Caesarean – if both babies are breech, or both babies are transverse (lying across the tummy), or if you've got a condition like placenta praevia, your twins share a placenta or you have had a difficult delivery with a single baby before you may well be advised to have a Caesarean. Some women really want to give birth vaginally and some feel happier about the idea of a Caesarean. It can depend on the mum's culture too. In some cultures and countries, a vaginal birth of twins would never be considered, so the mum might look at me in horror when I suggest it.

Q WHAT'S A GOOD SITUATION TO BE IN, FOR HAVING A VAGINAL BIRTH?

From an obstetrics point of view, we like the leading twin (the twin that is closest to the cervix) to be in a head-down position. We don't really mind what position the second twin is in, because the theory is that once twin one is born then twin two has suddenly got a lot of space in the uterus, and with the head being the heaviest part, gravity will push that baby into a head-down position. Sometimes, once twin one has already been born and the cervix is open, twin two can be successfully born in a breech position, but we would always prefer the second baby to be rotated into a head-down position.

Q WHEN WILL THE BIRTH BE DISCUSSED?

It will vary from area to area, but at the hospital I work at, generally speaking, we follow NICE guidance, so we start having a serious conversation about birth at around 28 weeks.

Q WHAT KINDS OF THINGS WILL AFFECT THE KIND OF BIRTH THAT IS RECOMMENDED?

We look at the positioning of the babies, your past obstetric history and if you've previously had a Caesarean we might recommend a Caesarean because a V-Bac (vaginal birth after Caesarean) can create issues with a twin pregnancy.

Q WHAT CAN I DO, TO BE FULLY INFORMED ON MY OPTIONS?

Check if your hospital runs parent education sessions where twin mums come along to talk about their experiences – they often get a mum who gave birth to twins vaginally and a mum who had a Caesarean to talk about why they went down that route If not, Twins Trust runs some great sessions where you can talk to twin mums about their births.

Q WHEN WILL THE BIRTH BE BOOKED FOR?

Again, it will vary slightly, but usually at the 32-week scan we start thinking about booking either an induction (if the babies are in a good position and you'd like a vaginal birth) or an elective Caesarean if the babies are in a poor position or you don't want to have a vaginal delivery. We'll book these in depending on the type of pregnancy it is – for a dichorionic pregnancy we recommend delivery between 37 and 38 weeks and for a monochorionic pregnancy, it's usually 36 to 37 weeks because we know that a placenta that is supplying two babies is going to mature more quickly than a placenta that's just supplying one baby.

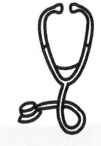

Q IS A HOME BIRTH OUT OF THE QUESTION?

Anything is possible! I think a lot of people think that health professionals are there to tell you what to do, but I really hope that's not the case. We're here to help you get what you want within the boundaries of safety. We usually recommend that you have your babies in the main unit of the hospital for many reasons – if you're being induced we'd need you in hospital because the induction process can't happen at home, and in an ideal world, we'd like to monitor the babies' heartbeats because they're at higher risk of becoming distressed than a singleton pregnancy and also your babies might need neonatal support. But if you know the risks and you're well informed, and you choose to have your twins at home, it's perfectly acceptable to try.

Q IF I'M HAVING A VAGINAL BIRTH, DO I HAVE TO BE INDUCED?

Absolutely not! In my experience, once you get to about 36 weeks, you might be saying: 'When can I have these babies?!' But if you feel great and the babies are growing well and you don't want to be induced then that is absolutely fine. You'd probably then be seen weekly for a scan to check that the placenta is still functioning well and to check the growth of the babies and so long as they are fine, you would be supported to continue until you go into spontaneous labour.

My postnatal care plan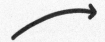

It's important to think about those first few weeks post-birth, as well as the actual birth, right now. Fill in the page opposite to form a plan for yourself . . .

THE PERSON (OR PEOPLE) WHO WILL
BE AROUND TO LOOK AFTER ME ARE:

I'M HAPPY/NOT HAPPY FOR VISITORS
IN THE FIRST FEW WEEKS

I CAN ASK FRIENDS
TO DO THE FOLLOWING
FOR ME:

3 MEALS I CAN
COOK AHEAD OF
TIME AND
FREEZE:

1

2

3

TREATS THAT I
CAN STOCK UP ON
AHEAD OF TIME:

6 THINGS you can do to prepare for your twin birth

Sophie Burch (@themammacoach)
birth coach and twin mum

1 Try hypnobirthing or antenatal hypnotherapy

Hypnobirthing classes are available nationwide and are a great way to learn breathing, visualisation and mindfulness techniques to help you in labour. Whether it's a class you attend or you download audiobooks or podcasts, it's such a good way to prepare for your twin birth. (Read more on page 106.) Antenatal hypnotherapy is a more tailored session aimed at meeting your individual needs. There are so many things that it can help with – confidence building, fear release, getting you feeling empowered, making you feel comfortable, helping you feel a lot calmer. It can help you visualise your birth and teach you about the use of language – how you talk to yourself to help you feel better.

2 Use mindfulness daily throughout your pregnancy

It's great to get into practice with mindfulness every day. I don't mean sitting and being like a Buddha, more just having a mindful approach to daily life. It's all about being in the present and being aware of your environment. From sensory things like what you're putting into your body, how it tastes, what does it smell like? To activities – what are you doing at the moment? Where are you sitting? What does it look like around you? When you're having a walk, it's about noticing the sounds around you and noticing what your environment looks like. When you are focusing on the present it prevents the mind from going back into the past and worrying about things, and stops us from thinking about the future – all the what ifs and whys and the things we have no control over. If you can practise this during pregnancy, it's something that can really help when your twins arrive. There will be so much going on all the time, so it's good to take stock, take time and give your mind a bit of stillness – even if it's just taking that moment to savour those first few sips of a cup of tea.

Be as open-minded as possible about your birth

I know that can be hard when you have your heart set on your birth being a certain way, but try to have a plan A, B and C, rather than having just one plan for your birth.

Write down your birth plan

Write down how you feel about your birth and your plans – A, B and C. Try to almost take an 'observer's view' – you can be so absorbed in all the possibilities that could happen during the birth that the fear kicks in and debilitates you. Whereas if you put the reality down on paper, then at least you can feel like you're being proactive again, and it can

allow you to feel more in control.

Reframe your worst-case scenario

It can be helpful to write down the worst-case scenario and reframe it. So, if your worst-case scenario is having a Caesarean section, what are the benefits to you? What are the benefits to the babies? And focus on the good things that can happen, so that might be having your babies on you straight away for skin to skin.

Choose a birth partner who can advocate for you

Make sure you have someone who is really prepared to ask questions, who knows what questions to ask, and knows how to create an environment that's conducive to you feeling good. During the birth, you're potentially not going to be in a place where you can communicate well. You might go into a state of fear and be unable to say all of the things that you want to say, and then regret it later. So it's important to have someone there who can do this for you.

Hypnobirthing

I loved doing hypnobirthing classes. The logic of it (by relaxing your body and reducing the stress hormones cortisol and adrenaline labour should be easier) makes a lot of sense to me. If you're a bit cynical about it, read up on the science it's based on, but also, just going to the classes or listening to hypnobirthing on audio can be a lovely, relaxing activity for you and your partner. Siobhan Miller (@shivy_miller), founder of The Positive Birth Company, shares her favourite breathing exercises for you to get started . . .

Breathing techniques to make your birth more positive

Siobhan Miller, The Positive Birth Company

Breathing is easy to do, it's completely free and you can do it anywhere. It's also the single most effective thing you can do to make your birth more positive. By following these simple breathing techniques you are ensuring you are bringing oxygen into your body (good for your muscles, which are working hard and good for your baby) and you're also keeping your heart rate steady and preventing yourself from getting into a panic, hyperventilating and producing adrenaline (aka the enemy of a good birth!).

I teach **two simple breathing techniques** – up-breathing and down-breathing. Up-breathing is for when your uterus muscles are drawing *upwards* and your cervix is dilating (the first stage of labour) and the down-breathing is for when your uterus muscles are pushing *downwards* and your baby descends and is born (the second stage).

Up-breathing:

Inhale slowly through your nose for a count of four, feel your chest expand and think to yourself 'inhale peace'. Then exhale slowly through your mouth for a count of eight, feeling your body soften and relax and think to yourself 'exhale tension'. Repeat four times.

Typically, once labour is established, a contraction lasts about 45 seconds to one minute, which means four reps of the 'in for four, out for eight' breathing pattern will have you covered. Once you complete the last exhale, the contraction will have passed and you'll know you're one step closer to meeting your babies!

This breathing technique can be used for any type of birth in any setting (including theatre) and indeed at any point in life when you want to feel a little calmer and more grounded.

Down-breathing:

You'll know when the time is right as you will feel your muscles pushing powerfully downwards. The sensation at first is not dissimilar to the feeling of needing a poo! So take a deep breath in through your nose, expanding your chest, and then exhale through your mouth but instead of a slow gentle exhale, channel your breath downwards through your body in a focused way. It's not forced pushing but it's using your exhale with intent. As you exhale in this way you will feel your stomach muscles engage and everything moving downwards in the right direction. What you want to do here is release all tension and HELP your body to birth your babies and not get in the way by tensing, drawing up and making it more difficult for them to descend and be born.

'I had two sets of twins – and planned two very different sets of birth!'

VICTORIA, MUM TO SEVEN-YEAR-OLD IDENTICAL TWINS, THREE-YEAR-OLD SINGLETON AND ONE-YEAR-OLD IDENTICAL TWINS

———

I've got two sets of twins and my experiences of planning the births were very different. During my first twin pregnancy, from an early stage, I was told that a planned C-section would be the best way forward but that if everything was looking OK, I could have a highly monitored vaginal birth. I was a little crushed that my ideal plans of a water birth were scuppered but I was keen to give my babies the safest entrance to the world possible and felt I had to trust the experts' opinions. I'd hear friends, who were due at a similar time, talking about water births, birth plans and midwife-led births. I found it upsetting that my birth would be largely out of my hands.

From 20 weeks onwards, at every fortnightly scan, I would enquire about what my chances of delivering naturally were. I was hopeful in the latter stages of my pregnancy because they told me both twins were presenting head down and I willed them to stay that way! I was told that under no circumstances would they let me go past the 37-week mark as the risks for identical twins sharing a placenta increased past this stage. I'd had no problems up to then but agreed to be induced at 37 weeks, even though I didn't really want to. I was told that I wouldn't be allowed to go into the birthing pool as they would need to check the babies on the ECG monitor. It seemed pointless voicing what I wanted as the day approached, because everything I wanted was deemed too risky. While I could understand the risks were greater than a singleton pregnancy, I still felt that I was largely not being heard. I guess I got used to saying yes to whatever they suggested and found my voice getting quieter and quieter, while inside I wanted to scream. In the end, I had to have a C-section because after five days of them trying to induce me in different ways, labour wasn't starting as it should and one of the twins was in distress. It was a world away from my original ideal birth scenario.

With my second set of twins I went about things very differently. I'd had a singleton baby in between, so I was lucky to have experience on my side and also the advice of an amazing midwife I met during my second pregnancy. The hospital pressed for me to have a C-section at 35 weeks, which I was massively opposed to. I was keen to have another V-Bac, but I was deemed even higher risk this time.

I made a very clear birth plan, where I wrote down things not just about the birth but about my surroundings and the terminology people used. I wanted the room to be kept dark and quiet, I asked for the clock to be removed, I requested that a minimal number of staff be present unless there was an emergency. I asked to be spoken to directly rather than for questions to be passed through my husband. I wanted minimal medical intervention unless it was entirely necessary. I was so sure of what I wanted and felt that I shouldn't be treated differently just because I was having twins. I was eager to have my views heard. My plans conflicted with what my consultant was advising so I arranged a meeting with the hospital's lead midwife for women-centred care. She reassured me and suggested I had a tour of the birthing rooms and meet some of the other midwives. The consultant wasn't happy with my decision but the birth went to plan. I was happy that I'd stuck to my plan and not just gone along with the consultant's wishes.

What to **PACK** in your hospital bag

You might have a date for a C-section or induction, or you might be waiting to go into labour spontaneously, but either way, it's wise to have your hospital bag packed and ready as early as you can. Here's what to pack for a twin birth . . .

FOR YOU

- ☐ Your birth plan and maternity notes
- ☐ A few nighties or PJs (Nighties are better after a C-section and buttons make feeding easier)
- ☐ Comfy joggers and T-shirt for going home
- ☐ Slippers
- ☐ Sanitary towels or stretchy disposable incontinence pants
- ☐ Big cotton knickers that will stretch over any potential C-section area (I still wear mine now – so comfy)
- ☐ Twin breastfeeding pillow
- ☐ Toiletries
- ☐ Hairband
- ☐ Snacks
- ☐ Water bottle
- ☐ Phone charger
- ☐ Peppermint teabags (really useful for shifting trapped wind after a C-section)

FOR THE BABIES

- ☐ Vests and sleepsuits (pack 10–15 of each – more than you think, in case you're in hospital for longer than you expect)
- ☐ Hats
- ☐ Blankets x 4 (two for each baby)
- ☐ Nappies
- ☐ Wipes/cotton wool
- ☐ Muslins (lots)
- ☐ Infant car seats

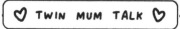

'I planned for a vaginal home birth experience'

ELLIE, MUM TO FOUR-YEAR-OLD NON-IDENTICAL TWINS
AND A SINGLETON, AGED EIGHT

I was keen to have a vaginal home birth, but as soon as two tiny beating hearts showed up on my dating scan, it became clear it was something I'd have to fight for. 'That's your home birth out of the window then!' commented the first midwife we saw as we sat still reeling from the shock.

Next came our appointment with our consultant, because of course we were now considered to be high-risk. We were told I would be induced at 36 weeks, given an epidural immediately upon arrival 'just in case', and that if I chose to refuse induction I would be 'no longer supported' by the hospital. I came away from the appointment feeling defeated. Luckily, a friend told me about a private midwife who could help. Unluckily, my fight continued and every admission to hospital included a battle, explaining why I was not under the Trust's care.

A week before I went into labour my private midwife cleared me for a home birth. When I went into labour and got into the birthing pool it wasn't long before the first twin – my daughter – made an appearance. It was amazing and so empowering! My son was born and needed some assistance breathing, so an ambulance was called, but he recovered quickly and had skin to skin with me while our daughter had skin to skin with her dad. I felt so relaxed and happy to be in my own surroundings, and so well cared for by the midwives.

Birth debriefs

Something I did to prepare for my twin birth was having a birth debrief. If this isn't your first pregnancy, I recommend you look into them.

When I was in the first trimester, a midwife friend told me about birth debriefs. I'd never heard of them and I hadn't been offered one after the birth of my eldest. 'I think you'll find it really helpful,' my friend said to me, over dinner. 'They'll get your birth notes and they'll talk you through what happened, the decisions that were made and the timings of everything. Some people find it a really good way of processing the experience, and if there's anything you're carrying guilt over it can help you see why things happened the way they did.' So I spoke to my midwife who arranged a birth debrief for me.

It was so helpful. We sat down and went through my birth notes, in chronological order. Thankfully, there was a box of tissues on the table next to us because it was a strangely emotional experience. Hearing the timings of things and reliving all the little developments and conversations that had happened felt strange. So many memories came flooding back. But it was so great to have someone to talk to about why certain decisions were made – and also to hear about how things have changed since then. There's now a much bigger focus on bladder health and midwives work closely with the urology team to look after a mum's bladder, so I was told that these days they'd have kept a closer eye on how often I was going to the loo during labour, which would probably have prevented the need for a catheter.

It was a cathartic and comforting experience and left me feeling a bit empowered – like, whatever my twin birth threw at me, I'd take it on and we'd get through it.

IF YOU ONLY DO 3 THINGS

1 Think about the kind of birth you'd like and discuss this at your next antenatal appointment.

2 Check if your hospital offers twin antenatal classes or workshops.

3 Plan what your postnatal care looks like.

Chapter 9

The birth *Fanfare*

As the date of my Caesarean section drew closer I felt two main emotions: relief that I'd made it to 36 weeks when the prospect of going into labour early with twins is a real possibility, and excitement about meeting my twin babies. It was comforting to know the date that (all being well) my twin birth would happen on. Maybe it's the control freak in me but I really liked having a date to work towards. From a practical point of view we could arrange for my mum to come and stay and look after our daughter while we were in the hospital, but also from an emotional point of view, it felt a lot easier.

Whether it's your first birth or you're adding to your family, it's a *huge moment*. It's life changing in so many ways! Not knowing when that huge life-changing moment will happen is something that I found tough when I had my first daughter. I spent day after day, heavily pregnant, pottering around the house trying to take my mind off the *one thing* that I was thinking about . . .

'Will today be the day my babies are born?'

. . . nevermind the added pressure of friends and family members helpfully enquiring by text.

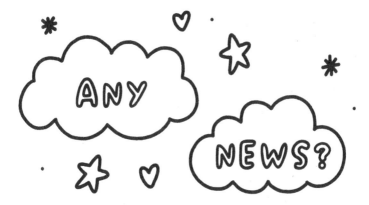

So with my twin pregnancy, having a date circled in my diary with 'C-section booked in' brought me some comfort. (Looking at my diary, now, I also had Robin from Hillary's Blinds booked in to come over that afternoon, and frankly, I think I had slightly unrealistic expectations of the day. What did I think was going to happen? Have the babies in the morning and be home in time to have the new blinds fitted at 4pm?!)

The days in the lead up to the *big day* were a flurry of seeing friends for a cuppa (one last time before the babies arrive!) and doing last minute sorting of things – washing newborn clothing, building a chest of drawers for them to go in, buying giant black postpartum knickers – and everyday admin like taking library books back ('If I don't do it now, I'll never have time and imagine the late fees!' I stressily told my husband).

A few days before my C-section date I had to visit the hospital to have bloods taken and to have two steroid injections. Now, I imagine this is different in every hospital, but at mine they make you come to the Maternity Assessment Unit, which is in the labour ward. It was the same labour ward that I'd had my daughter in eight years previously and just walking down the corridors to the ward triggered all sorts of difficult memories that I'd been suppressing.

They popped me into a bay with a bed and the curtains drawn shut, where I waited for a midwife to become available to tend to me. In the nextdoor bay a lady was in labour and I could hear her having contractions and being talked through it all by her mum.

I sat there, anxiety flooding through me, suddenly feeling tearful and wobbly at the idea of giving birth in a few days' time. 'It's OK,' I told myself, 'I'm going to be fine. I'm having a C-section, it's going to be different this time.'

I know that for many women having a vaginal birth is the ideal, but I knew that my mental health couldn't take it, and this experience confirmed that having a Caesarean was, without a doubt, the best thing I could be doing.

By the time the midwife came along to give me the steroid injection in my bum (which – heads up – is painful!) I felt much calmer.

On the morning of the birth we got up early, kissed our daughter goodbye and headed off to the hospital for 7am. I wasn't allowed to eat anything ahead of the procedure and as we arrived at the hospital and got checked in my tummy was already rumbling.

We were taken to a bay in a room earmarked for mums having Caesareans and people came in and out to take my blood pressure and ask questions. The oddest moment was when someone popped in to shave some of my pubic hair off! I mean, I could have done that at home if I'd known it needed to be done!? But there's no point in having any kind of 'shame' when you're giving birth, is there? Whether it's bodily functions, flashing your bits or having someone you've only just met come at you with an electric shaver, it's all good, right?

We were given regular updates on where we were on the list of procedures. We started off as being first in the queue, because we were having twins, but a couple of emergency C-sections came in so by the time it was our turn it was 1.30pm.

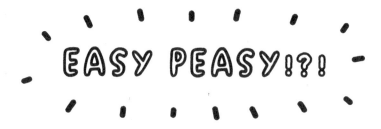

EASY PEASY!?!

Walking into the operating theatre was such a surreal experience – after all, you don't usually see inside them, do you? Previously when I've had operations I've been under anaesthetic before being wheeled into theatre.

The radio was on playing middle-of-the-road pop music and the room was filled with a lot of people – the anaesthetic team, midwives, a consultant obstetrician and paediatricians – and there were two of some of them because we were having twins. They were all busying about doing things in preparation and I had to sit on the edge of the operating table to have my epidural anaesthetic. My main memory of this was being given a very specific set of instructions that seemed impossible! 'I'd like you to curve your back, look down but try to relax and stay *very very* still,' the anaesthetist said to me. Easy peasy, right?! Shall I also stand on one leg and juggle those surgical instruments? Afterwards, she sprayed water on my tummy to test whether the anaesthetic had worked, and it had. Phew!

Next, a blue curtain went up between my head and my abdomen and they started the procedure. My husband – dressed in scrubs – stayed at the head end with me. 'I'm not sure I want to see what happens,' he smiled nervously at me.

As they got started with the procedure the anaesthetist chatted to me, asking me questions to take my mind off things and also updating me on what was happening. 'They've made the first incision,' she said calmly, as if she was describing being able to see a relaxing spa treatment in progress. I could feel myself shaking and couldn't stop myself. I assumed it was a nervous reaction but it was explained to me that it's a common reaction to the anaesthetic.

I could feel a bit of movement in my abdominal area, but nothing painful or uncomfortable and before I knew it the anaesthetist was saying, 'They've got the first baby out!' and I could see her being held up above the blue curtain for us to see *Lion King*-style! It was such an emotional yet surreal moment – to have your baby held up for you to clap eyes on for the first time ever. 'Now, they're going to get the second baby but sometimes this can take a bit longer because the baby suddenly has a lot more room in there so they can move away from us,' explained the anaesthetist. It was so helpful having her calmly explain what was going on.

At that moment, I glanced up and realised that the large surgical light above me had a very reflective metallic surface and if I wasn't careful I'd be able to see what was happening reflected back at me!

After a few minutes the second baby was out and being held up for us to see. While they got busy stitching me up, the babies were checked over and wrapped up before being brought over for us to have a closer look. The whole experience was exactly what I needed it to be – calm, efficient and importantly, totally different to my previous birth.

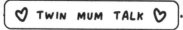

'I had a vaginal twin birth and no induction'

EMMA, MUM TO IDENTICAL TWINS, AGED FIVE

When I discovered I was pregnant, I was immediately keen to give birth at home. I'd had a baby already and with that birth there was a lot of intervention: epidural, episiotomy and ventouse, so I wanted a home birth this time. When I found out I was having twins, I realised this was unlikely.

I was 34 weeks pregnant when I discussed birth options with the consultant and explained that my preferences were a vaginal birth with as little intervention as possible. I didn't want a cannula or an epidural, I didn't want to be tied to a bed, I didn't want to give birth on my back. The consultant wasn't happy about my wishes and made me feel like I was asking for something quite dangerous. So I found a local doula, booked an hour with her and she talked me through what a more natural twin birth could look like. It gave me the confidence to go back to the hospital and question what they were saying.

I was 36 weeks plus six and my waters broke at 2am. I went to hospital at 4am and everything was done by 5.30am. I gave birth to Henry on all fours on the bed and then they turned me around and 14 minutes later I gave birth to Ben.

I felt so lucky that it had all gone to plan – it couldn't have gone any better, really. The recovery was quick – I was up and about very quickly, as if nothing had happened! I'm so glad I pushed for a vaginal delivery with as little intervention as possible.

WHAT TO EXPECT FROM A VAGINAL TWIN DELIVERY

* **If you're booked in for an induction**, labour will be artificially started by a vaginal pessary or gel of prostaglandin, which softens the cervix. If that doesn't bring on labour, you might have your waters broken and if that still doesn't get things going, the third thing they'll do is put you on an oxytocin drip.

* **If you choose to wait for labour to begin naturally** you'll let the hospital know when your contractions begin and they'll let you know when to come in.

* **You might want pain relief** while you wait for labour to progress and as the contractions get stronger – epidurals are often recommended for twin births.

* **When you're fully dilated and ready to give birth** you might be moved to an operating theatre, or you might be allowed to stay in the delivery suite.

* **If it's taking longer than usual** for the first twin to be born forceps or ventouse might be suggested to help things along.

* **Once twin one is born, gravity should encourage twin two to move into a head-down position** but sometimes having all that extra room means they can get themselves into an awkward position. When this happens you might need obstetric help to stabilise the baby and move it to a head-down position.

* **If twin two is taking a long time to be born** you might be offered a hormone drip to encourage the birth.

* **The final stage of labour is delivering the placenta** (or placentas if you have two) and you'll be offered an injection of Syntocinon or Syntometrine to speed up the contraction of the uterus and the delivery of the placenta. You don't have to have this injection but it's often recommended for twin births.

HOW ARE YOU FEELING?

Whether you've given birth vaginally before or not, waiting to go into labour can be a pretty intense time. If you're being induced, as the date of the induction approaches you might be feeling apprehensive, nervous and scared . . . or you might have bubbles of excitement in your tummy, ready to experience this incredibly awesome thing – giving birth to your two babies! Basically, there is no right or wrong way to feel and you might be feeling a mix of all of the above.

Pessaries can take a while to work, so it's a good idea to have entertainment in your hospital bag – that can't-put-down novel you're reading and your tablet loaded up with episodes of *Gilmore Girls*.

If you're not being induced the wait to go into labour can feel like it's taking forever. Especially when you're carrying the weight of two babies! Take it easy in those final few days – trashy TV, lots of sofa time and getting fresh air when you can is a great idea.Think about what things might help keep you calm and feeling positive while you're in labour – it might be hypnobirthing tracks, a meditation podcast or it could be relaxing music. Check out the breathing exercises on page 106.

WHAT TO EXPECT FROM A C-SECTION

* **You'll be given steroid injections** a few days before the procedure to mature your babies' lungs and make it easier for them to breathe when they're born.

* **You won't be allowed to eat or drink for several hours** before the procedure.

* **You'll be given an epidural** – which means you won't be able to feel anything from the waist down, but you'll be awake throughout the procedure.

* **You'll also have an IV drip fitted to your arm** in case it's needed, and a catheter will be fitted and will stay in for around 24 hours.

* **The C-section will take place in an operating theatre.** A screen will be raised between your head and the procedure.

* **The obstetrician will make an incision** across your bikini line and the baby nearest to them will be removed first.

* **Sometimes the second twin can wriggle away** from the incision, so it can take a bit longer for that one to be born.

* **The babies will be checked over** while the obstetrician delivers the placenta(s) and stitches you back up.

HOW ARE YOU FEELING?

If you're booked in for a C-section it's understandable to feel nervous as the date gets nearer. It's major abdominal surgery, after all. But try to focus on the bigger picture – you'll get to meet your babies soon. You might be feeling very chilled about it if you've had a C-section before and know what to expect, or even if you haven't and know that it's the safest way for your babies to be born.

On the day of your Caesarean there might be a long wait before you're taken to theatre, so it can be a good idea to go armed with some magazines, a book or a film downloaded onto your tablet so that you don't spend the whole time pacing the room and obsessing over how hungry you are and how you could murder a cheese sandwich.

. . . *and* if the babies have to be delivered early

With all twin births there's a possibility that they might be born prematurely – before your planned induction or C-section date. Reasons for this include pre-eclampsia, high-blood pressure in the mum, vaginal bleeding, Twin to Twin Transfusion Syndrome and gestational diabetes.

It can be a really good idea to have a tour of the SCBU (Special Care Baby Unit) or NICU (Neonatal Intensive Care Unit) in your local hospital during your pregnancy. It can prepare you mentally for the possibility of having your babies in there receiving care when they're born.

'**I delivered one twin vaginally and the other twin by C-section**'

AMY, MUM TO TWO-YEAR-OLD TWINS

I planned to have a vaginal delivery and my consultant supported my decision, so I was induced at 37.5 weeks. It wasn't until my third day in the maternity ward, after the midwives decided to break my waters, that the contractions began.

Our first daughter was delivered at just before 7pm; we were able to have lots of immediate skin-to-skin contact and she latched onto the breast. I was so preoccupied with her that I had little awareness of what was going on in the room around me, but it soon became apparent there was a problem with the second twin. She had turned and was now lying in a transverse position.

It was explained to me that I would be taken into the operating theatre where they would initially try to turn the baby externally (ECV). My husband was by my side the whole time and our first twin was in her cot next to us. Almost an hour passed while the staff attempted to turn the second twin but in the end she refused to budge, so we went ahead and did a C-section. Although it was technically an 'emergency C-section', it never had that sense of stress or urgency. My advice to expectant twin mums is to be open-minded and expect the unexpected. Listen to the medical advice but do your own reading on birth options too. There is no right or wrong way to give birth; the safe arrival of your babies is all that matters.

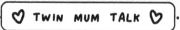

'I had a C-section twin birth'

ANDIE, MUM OF IDENTICAL 22-MONTH-OLD TWIN GIRLS

When I was 32 weeks we went for our weekly growth scan at the hospital and we were told I'd need to have a C-section within the next 24 hours. One of the babies had stopped growing and there were issues with blood flow. I'd had laser ablation surgery and amniotic fluid reduction at 20 weeks to deal with TTTS and every week the girls stayed inside after that was a bonus.

I went home to get my hospital bag, a pillow and blanket and then headed back to the hospital. The procedure didn't happen until 9.30pm – being unable to eat anything was torture! I thought I was mentally prepared for the Caesarean but when they wheeled me into theatre I started panicking and wanted to run away! Was it too late to change my mind?! I kept telling my partner I was scared. The nurses and doctors in the room were all being very blasé! They were talking and chatting like it was all very normal – which it obviously is to them, but to me it felt like I was watching a TV show.

I couldn't believe how quick the C-section was. When the girls were born they were rushed off to NICU and I didn't get to hold them or properly see them for five hours. But I was just so happy they were both alive after the struggle of TTTS. I had been told by my midwife that they'd probably be whisked off so we took a Polaroid camera into theatre and I asked the staff to take photos of the girls and I just stared at them until I finally got to meet them properly.

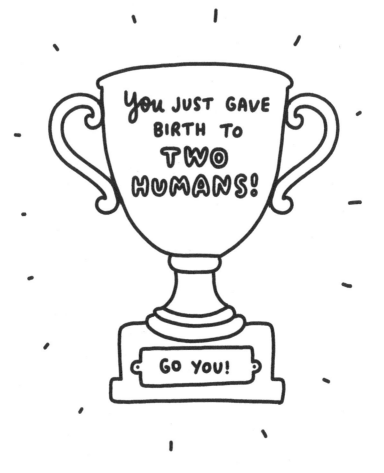

IF YOU ONLY DO 3 THINGS

1 Stay calm – you can handle whatever your twin birth throws at you.

2 Tell yourself how strong you are. You've grown two babies! You can give birth to them.

3 Remember your plans B and C (from Chapter 7).

Chapter 10

The first few days in hospital

There are a few times in my life when I wish I was on some fly-on-the-wall reality TV show and have video footage to scroll back through. You know, those moments that are big life moments but when you look back at them your memory is hazy or has huge empty pockets where you have no recollection of what happened. Wouldn't it be handy if you'd had two or three cameras recording it all from different angles and a nicely packaged programme to remind you? Gah, Kim Kardashian is so lucky!

When I think back now the first few hours after giving birth to my twins are a massive blur. My memory seems to skip from being in the operating theatre, seeing the twins for the first time to being back in the recovery room, but I have no recollection of being wheeled there on my hospital bed. Likewise, my memories of the next few hours are patchy – I remember eating a sandwich and (rather randomly) drinking some Fanta (I'd been looking forward to the famous 'tea and toast' that you so often hear about post-birth, but my local hospital had to ban toasters because they were setting off fire alarms too often!). We were told that the twins, who'd been born at 5lbs and 5lbs 2oz, were mostly fine – one needed to be popped under a lamp for a while to regulate her temperature – but other than that, all was good.

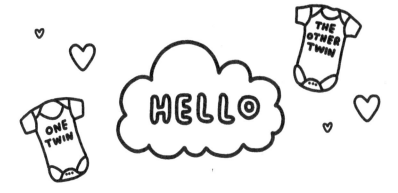

The midwives had put little home-knitted hats on them when they were first born and they were wrapped in blankets. I gave them skin to skin and tried breastfeeding them both. It was hard – they were both such sleepy little things. I just felt so relieved to have them here, safe and well. I'd been mentally preparing myself for them to be whisked off to SCBU, so to be told they were OK was such a huge relief.

I was moved to the regular maternity ward and soon after it was discovered that both twins had a problem with low blood-sugar levels, which can happen with babies born before 37 weeks. They had to have blood tests every three hours before being fed – it was awful hearing them cry as their tiny feet were pricked to get blood – and I was told we had to get the results over a certain level (above 2.6mmol/L). We had to get good results three tests in a row in order to be sure each baby's blood-sugar levels were OK.

At this point I still couldn't feel the lower half of my body because of the anaesthetic. It was starting to wear off slightly – I could feel a sensation if I touched my abdomen – but I couldn't move my legs. They were strapped into a piece of equipment that was a bit like a giant blood-pressure checker – every so often it would compress my legs and then release. I was aware – from giving birth once before at the same hospital – that dads weren't allowed to stay overnight, so at around 10pm I sent my husband home to get a good night's sleep. Which – in hindsight – was utter madness! There I was, lying in a hospital bed unable to move my legs or stand up, with two small newborn babies lying next to me, who I couldn't even lean over to pick up without help. I could hear, through the curtains separating me from the other new mums in the ward, that dads were still around through the night, so the rules must have been relaxed.

Thankfully, at around 2am, a midwife realised I was on my own (what she thought of us, I'll never know!). 'We're not too busy tonight,' she said to me, kindly. 'Why don't I take them with me, and let you get some sleep? I'll bring them back in a few hours when they need to be fed.' I could have kissed her. Her kindness – and common sense – allowed me to have a few hours' sleep, which as you might know, for any new mum is like gold dust.

The next morning the feeling in my legs had returned and I was told I was being moved to my own room. They explained that if there's space the hospital gives twin mums a private room because you're more likely to be there for a bit longer. I remembered the advice I'd read about getting up and about quickly after a C-section, so when the healthcare assistants came to move me I decided to try to get up and walk. Well! After three steps I nearly passed out from the pain!

Note to self: Take things a bit more slowly.

I allowed the staff to wheel me to my room in my bed. 'Any chance of some more painkillers?' I asked them, hopefully.

We were in hospital for four nights and five days in total, and those days were a bit of a blur of feeding, skin-to-skin cuddles, injecting myself with blood-thinning medication, changing nappies and people coming in and out of the room for myriad reasons.

<u>knock knock</u>
Hi! I'm here to test the babies' blood-sugar levels!
<u>knock knock</u>
Hi! I'm here to remove your catheter!
<u>knock knock</u>
Hi! I'm here to give you your medication and check your blood pressure!
<u>knock knock</u>
Hi! I'm here to check on how your tummy is healing!
<u>knock knock</u>
Hi! I'm here to give the babies their vitamin K injection!

Their what? This was total news to me – but it was explained that all newborns are offered this to help prevent a rare bleeding disorder called haemorrhagic disease of the newborn. Hopefully you're more clued up than I was!

<u>knock knock</u>
Hi! I'm here to give the babies their BCG immunisation!
<u>knock knock</u>
Hi! I'm here to give you your Bounty pack!

This lady got a swift, 'No thank you!' from me. Honestly, if I can give you one piece of advice from one mum to another, it's this: don't feel pressurised into buying photographs from, or handing over your email address to, the Bounty lady if she visits you – not all hospital trusts allow Bounty access to the maternity wards, but if yours does, you don't have to speak to her. The last thing any new mum – let alone a new twin mum – needs when she is recovering from giving birth is a salesperson approaching her in her bed. Thankfully, being in our own room, it was easy for my husband to stay with me overnight. There was even a chair that fully reclined so he could get some sleep.

Once the catheter was out the day after giving birth I decided to attempt to shuffle to the loo. With a lot of help from my husband, I managed it. I felt like a hero! For the five days I was in hospital every day I made myself get up a few times. I'd swing my legs slowly over the side of the bed, have to pause there and take some deep breaths, before gently standing up and hobbling to the loo. What felt like an impossible task on day two felt much easier by day three and four. On day four I even managed to shuffle all the way up the corridor to the tea trolley! Honestly, the feeling of elation was – I'm sure – akin to someone who'd just run a marathon. It was incredible how quickly the recovery was happening.

The day after the twins were born our eldest daughter came to meet her two brand-new sisters for the first time. She'd gone from being an only child for eight years to having two sisters! She felt like all her Christmases had come at once. 'Can I hold one?' she asked, her big eyes looking up at us with hope. We sat her down on the big chair, popped pillows on her knees to create a bit of a nest and placed one of the babies on her knee. 'I'm so happy but I also want to cry,' she said. Once she'd cuddled both babies, laid on the bed, eaten a picnic tea and helped get me a cuppa from the trolley it was time for her to go home. Introducing her to her little sisters was such a gorgeously special moment.

How long you should expect to be in hospital?

As with singleton babies, the discharge of twins is dependent on established feeding, hearing screening, clinical wellness and ensuring there's adequate support for the parents. The length of time you spend in hospital following your twin birth will depend on how straightforward your pregnancy and birth was and how your babies are doing in the first few hours and days. If your babies are doing well they'll be allowed to stay with you in the hospital ward (you might even be given your own room if there's one available and if you speak to the senior midwife, your partner might be able to stay longer than the usual visiting hours). If there are complications one or both of your babies might have to go to the hospital's Special Baby Care Unit (SCBU) or Neonatal Intensive Care Unit (NICU). Sometimes it's necessary to move to a different hospital if certain care is required. See page 138 for more on SCBU and NICU.

Some twins are discharged soon after birth, but often, issues like infection, jaundice, respiratory issues, blood sugar levels, feeding problems – and your recovery, too – might mean it's a few days or longer before you can go home with your babies. Even if you've had a straightforward birth, you may find that one or both of your babies has complications that need to be treated on the postnatal ward. You might also find that one twin is discharged but the other has to stay in hospital for longer, which can be emotionally and logistically tough when you're trying to care for both babies. See page 138 for more advice on this.

5 THINGS that might make you feel better in the first few days

Mars Lord (@_marslord), doula and twin mum

1 Skin to skin

As soon as you can, you should do skin to skin with your babies. This can really help you bond with your babies, so straight after the delivery is a great time. More and more hospitals are allowing skin to skin after a Caesarean. Find out what the hospital means by skin to skin, for some it's the baby's cheek touching you. But ideally, skin to skin means as much of your skin and the baby's skin touching as possible. Theatre's quite cold, so they might only allow you a few minutes of skin to skin before they send you off to recovery, where hopefully you can tuck the babies in beside you. Midwives and doctors can be obsessed with babies being cold, but during skin to skin, your core temperature goes up if the babies are cold and your core temperature goes down if the babies are too hot. If you can't do skin to skin, then get your partner to do it. Or have a baby each and then swap over.

2 Try to get proper breastfeeding support

Most midwives either don't have specialist breastfeeding knowledge or, even if they do, they don't have time to sit with every new mum. So it can be a really good idea, before the birth, to speak to a lactation consultant or do a breastfeeding class (see page 148 for more) to learn about how breastfeeding twins works. Ask if the hospital has a breastfeeding specialist – particularly an IBCLC (International Board Certified Lactation Consultant) and find out when they visit the hospital.

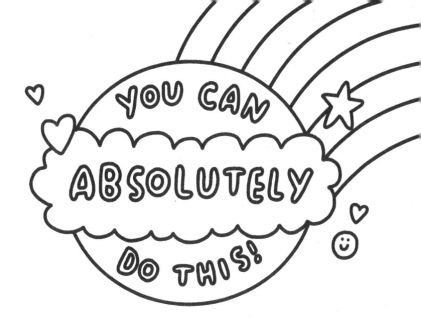

YOU CAN
ABSOLUTELY
DO THIS!

3 If you feel overwhelmed, stop and breathe

One of my favourite sayings is 'How do we eat an elephant? One bite at a time.' It's easy to sit there and feel overwhelmed by having two small babies to feed and care for, but just think of one thing that needs doing – then do that. Then think of another – then do that. Take things one at a time

4 Tell yourself: You can do this

One of the main reasons I'm hired as a doula for twins is that people tell me I'm the first person they've met who's positive about twins. People hear: 'Oh, it's twins, well you'll have to have a Caesarean, you won't be able to breastfeed, you'll need to get a nanny, you won't get any sleep, you've got to get them into a routine or they'll destroy you.' It's other people's fear of the unknown. But you can do this.

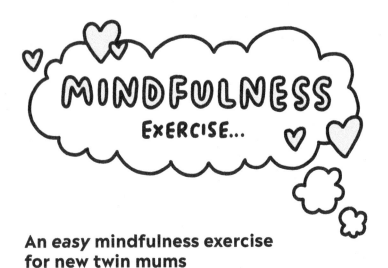

An *easy* mindfulness exercise for new twin mums

As discussed earlier in the book (see page 104), mindfulness is a great way to stop and take note of what's happening around you. Training your brain to be in the present moment helps to alleviate anxiety.

Next time you are doing skin to skin with your babies, tune in to your senses.

* **How does their skin feel against yours?**
* **What do their heads smell of?**
* **Are they making any little snuffling noises?**

Registering all of this could boost your oxytocin levels. Oxytocin is a hormone (known as 'the love hormone') which is released when you have skin-to-skin contact with your babies and breastfeed. It lowers stress levels (in you and the babies) and creates a bond between mum and babies.

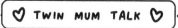

'I felt like Superwoman in the first few days!'

HARRIET, MUM TO TWO-YEAR-OLD TWINS

My birth was amazing! In the days and weeks that followed I felt like Superwoman. After they'd been born, I remember being very disorientated and going from watching my mum and husband with my children while I was stitched up to suddenly having them plonked on my chest as I was wheeled to the ward. I ate a lot of toast – I think the midwives must have toasted a whole loaf of bread for me!

The next day, Gwen wasn't feeding brilliantly and it was picked up that she had jaundice. A doctor inserted a nasogastric tube and she had to spend 24 hours having light therapy, which was unbelievably hard because we couldn't pick her up.

We thought we'd get to go home the next day, but by this point both of the babies had lost over 10 per cent of their body weight. We were moved to the ward next door where there was an amazing midwife who asked us how we felt about bottle-feeding her, an opportunity we jumped at. My husband completely broke down when he was able to feed his daughter for the first time and it'll always be a very special memory for me. Frustratingly, we were on that ward for longer than we'd hoped because every time Gwen put on weight, Dorothy would lose it and vice versa. When we were finally given the OK to be discharged, six days after the girls were born, it was amazing. When we left, we honestly felt like naughty children or like we'd just broken out of prison!

If your babies need special care . . .

Of course, it's not always so easy in the first few days. It's common for twins to have to spend some time in SCBU if they're very small and need extra care, like oxygen, treatment for low blood sugar or having their breathing or heart rate monitored. Some have to go NICU if they're particularly premature, unwell and need specialised care. According to Twins Trust, 40 per cent of multiples need some kind of extra care when they're born.

It can be a really tough time emotionally to have one, or both, of your twins needing special care – you might feel helpless or worried. Having one or both babies in a special unit, perhaps with tubes and incubators, can feel daunting and a world away from how you imagined your first few days with them would be.

My advice for you if one, or both, twins are in SCBU or NICU

Pam Langford, multiple birth specialist midwife, East and North Hertfordshire NHS Trust

 Try to get involved in the daily routine care
Actively participate, ask to change the nappies, do the nasal gastric tube feeds. We encourage breastfeeding as the babies tolerate it better when they are premature. (They find formula difficult to digest and can spend a lot of energy that's needed for growing digesting formula. In theory, this speeds up the process of coming home.)

SKIN TO SKIN

Always ask for the babies to be given to you skin to skin (*also known as kangaroo care*)

This is really important for the babies' wellbeing, they experience the smell of their parent and it enhances breastfeeding cues and encourages breastmilk production. You might have to prompt NICU to help with this, they can sometimes be busy and it's tricky when babies are caught up in wires etc. The benefit to the babies far outweighs the effort to remove the babies from the incubators.

Constant communication

Doctors carry out regular rounds in NICU. They discuss the previous 24 hours of your babies' time in NICU. This includes feeds, nappies, medications, breathing requirements and baby observation. They then build a forward plan for their care based on the findings. Try to ensure that you are available on the unit at this set time to be able to listen to what is said. Being present allows transparency and builds relationships with the team. Parents report that they feel actively involved in their babies' care, the parents' mental health seems to benefit from this and they retain 'ownership' of their children. They have fewer trauma symptoms and more positive affirmations around the babies.

'My babies spent four weeks in SCBU'

MICHELLE, MUM TO 16-MONTH-OLD TWINS

My babies were born at 31 weeks and 3 days. They allowed my partner to take a few pictures for me, but then they were put into what I can only describe as looking like a vacuum pack bag, obviously not to catch any germs, and taken to NICU. It was such a big shock to my system. I've never felt as low or cried as much. I didn't get to see my babies for four hours after they were born, and when I did finally see them, in incubators, it was heart-breaking.

The next day they were moved out of intensive care and into the high-dependency unit. The first time I got to hold them and do skin to skin was the best feeling ever. We couldn't hold them too much as they needed to be in the incubators as much as possible, but when I did, it was simply the best. After eight nights, the babies were transferred to a different hospital where they were in SCBU for three weeks. I'd been expressing breastmilk and the babies were being tube fed but in Special Care they let us be involved in every aspect and trained us to tube feed our babies.

No one prepares you for having premature babies and the emotional rollercoaster it brings. I blamed myself – was it the bath salts I used? Maybe I had meat that wasn't cooked well enough? – all of this goes through your head. I felt angry, guilty, sad and at times lonely. But if your babies are in SCBU, try to think of the positives – our time there got us into a really good routine, which made things much easier at home.

MY MINI POST-BIRTH JOURNAL

I'M PROUD OF MYSELF BECAUSE...

THINGS I FEEL GRATEFUL FOR RIGHT NOW...

THINGS I NEED RIGHT NOW...

Self-care for twin mums with babies in SCBU or NICU . . .

Mars Lord (@_marslord), doula and twin mum shares her advice

 Think about who's going to look after you
You're going to be using up all your energy and time concentrating on your babies in SCBU or NICU, so you need someone to be your support. Who's going to make sure you're fed and watered?

 If you can, get them on your skin as much as possible
Spend as much time as possible in SCBU with them. You don't have to go away to your hospital bed and rest for hours. You can rest by sitting in a chair in SCBU with your babies on your skin. So often mums are told, 'I'll call you when it's time to feed them,' but spending time with your babies is valuable and you can rest while you do it.

 That said, work out when you're going to sleep
Perhaps your partner can sit with the babies – and do skin to skin – while you're back in your bed having a sleep. And then you can swap. But it's important you get enough rest.

IF YOU ONLY DO 3 THINGS

1 Get as much skin to skin with your babies as you can - it helps with bonding, breastfeeding and boosting your oxytocin (known as 'the love hormone').

2 If you feel overwhelmed, stop and breathe.

3 Get as much rest as you can.

Chapter 11

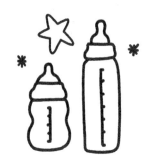

Feeding your twins

'Will you breastfeed them?'

'You can't breastfeed twins, can you?'

'How on earth does breastfeeding twins work?'

'If you feed them one at a time won't you just constantly be breastfeeding them in the early days?'

'Breastfeeding two? When will you get time to go to the loo or have a sandwich?!'

There are so many preconceptions around feeding twins – you'll probably have heard some of the above. And, as with all babies, there's no right or wrong way to feed them. If they've been born prematurely, or need extra help in SCBU or NICU, your babies might need to be fed in a certain way (using cups, tubes or bottles) but otherwise, how you feed your babies is your choice.

And it's totally possible to breastfeed twins, if that's what you choose.

I breastfed my first daughter – back then I'd had an open mind and thought, 'I'll give it a go and see what happens,' but I didn't put any pressure on myself. I knew that breastfeeding was considered the best way to feed your baby for so many reasons, but I also knew that a lot of mums struggle with it. As it happened, after a bit of a painful, tricky start, we got into the rhythm of it and I breastfed her until she was six months old.

So when I was pregnant with my twins, and people asked me: 'Will you breastfeed them?' I had exactly the same approach. I knew I'd managed to breastfeed my first daughter, but that was no guarantee that I'd manage it this time, and . . . there would be two of them! I decided to give breastfeeding a go and see what happened.

After giving birth I hadn't been in the recovery bay for long at all before a lady appeared offering to help get some colostrum out of my breasts. I later discovered she was part of the hospital's Infant Feeding Team (something that some hospital trusts have – it's worth finding out ahead of your birth whether your hospital has one), and in what went down as another utterly bizarre experience, she helped massage my breasts in a way that allowed her to collect tiny droplets of colostrum from my nipples with a pipette. The colostrum was then given to the babies. She taught me how to do it myself and she also helped me put the babies on the breast, showing me how to wake them up by blowing on them or tickling under their chins. I did lots of skin to skin with the babies to encourage the milk production and it was just lovely.

Over the next few days the support we got from the Infant Feeding Team in hospital was incredible. There was always one person on duty, so we could call for help or she would pop her head in to see how we were getting on. We were feeding the twins every three hours – the biggest struggle was getting them to stay awake! They were such sleepy little things and after a little bit of feeding they'd zonk out again.

On the second day the Infant Feeding Team were a bit concerned about the babies' weights, so they suggested we top up the breastfeeds with formula. They gave us tiny bottles and a cold-water steriliser, and my husband took on the job of organising the washing and sterilising of the bottles. He also helped me to bottle-feed the babies after each breastfeed. It was really lovely for him to have a proper role in those early days, and to be able to help feed his new daughters.

Then it was suggested that I could express breast milk and that it could encourage my milk flow. The hospital staff gave me a heavy-duty electric breast pump, showed me how to use it and I got into a routine of breastfeeding the babies, topping up with some formula and then expressing milk, which I'd give to them on the next feed (this is sometimes called 'triple feeding'). For me, this all worked because I was doing the best I could for my babies – working on cracking breastfeeding them, helping my milk flow increase – but I was also ensuring they were getting enough milk by topping up with formula. I didn't feel even a small iota of guilt for doing things this way – I feel so strongly that every baby is different, every mum is different, and we all just have to do what we think is best for ourselves, our babies and our family.

One benefit of being in hospital for five days was having that feeding support 24/7. Support varies from hospital to hospital but I was fortunate to have a really dedicated team of feeding experts on hand. They showed me how to position pillows in a way that allowed me to tandem feed the twins at the same time, which I carried on doing for the ten months that I breastfed them.

It helped to keep a log of feeds. We scribbled down in a notebook for each twin the time they fed, how long they'd breastfed for, how much expressed milk they'd had and how much formula they'd had. With my foggy, sleep-deprived brain it really helped to have a log when we were asked how the last couple of feeds had gone.

Write THE names OF THE
PEOPLE IN THIS CIRCLE WHOSE
BUSINESS IT IS
HOW YOU FEED
YOUR TWINS...

(CLUE: THERE SHOULD JUST
BE YOUR NAME AND YOUR
TWINS' NAMES IN THE CIRCLE)

7 TIPS to help you breastfeed your twins

Kathryn Stagg, international board certified lactation consultant who specialises in multiple birth families

1 Surround yourself with positive, breastfeeding mums!

You might find that friends, family and even health professionals can be very negative about breastfeeding more than one baby. So you can benefit greatly from surrounding yourself with positive people and connecting with others that have done it before. This is where Twins Groups, specialist antenatal sessions and social media are really useful.

2 Search out your local breastfeeding support

Find your local International Board Certified Lactation Consultant. You can even make contact before the babies arrive. I am often contacted by expectant mums wanting to make sure I will be available around their birth date. Find your local breastfeeding peer supporters for emotional support and more basic breastfeeding support. Google will tell you most of this, but also ask your midwife, health visitor and local mums what is available near you.

3 Ask for help

Ask for as much help as you can when you're in hospital with your twins. But it's important to remember that breastfeeding is a thing you and your babies will learn together and improve with practice. We can learn the theory before the babies arrive, but it is not until they are actually here that you can really know what it's all about. Some babies and mums get it straight away; for others it can take a little while to come together. But the most important thing is to keep the babies fed, keep the milk flowing and keep the babies close because then you will have options.

Remember 'triple feeding' is hard work but only temporary

Twin babies are often born a little earlier, smaller and more sleepy than your average newborn. So many families find themselves 'triple feeding' to begin with. Triple feeding is when the babies are not feeding efficiently enough to fully breastfeed and so they need to be topped up a little in the early days. Then mum needs to pump to protect her milk supply. It is a lot of hard work but the good news is that it's temporary and once babies are around due date and a bit more alert you can move towards exclusive breastfeeding if you wish.

Try tandem feeding before being discharged from hospital

This doesn't mean that you need to do it all the time when you get home, but it's very empowering as a new mum of twins to know that you can feed two at the same time. It takes a lot of the stress out of the situation when they are both crying. Some prefer to tandem feed from the start, others wait a bit, others only do it sometimes and others don't like it and so rarely do it. It's completely individual!

 Aim for a minimum of eight feeds in 24 hours

In the early days a good plan to stick to is feeding them every three hours from the start of each feed. But once the babies begin to consistently wake before that time and nappy output and weight gain is good, then it can be a good idea to move towards responsive feeding.

Don't worry if one twin feeds better than the other

It's very common for this to happen in the early days. It is so important to remember they are individuals. Specialist breastfeeding support will be able to help get a deeper latch and better positioning if you need it, but sometimes it is just a waiting game and one baby can take a bit longer to get it.

4 WAYS to breastfeed your twins

There are a few different tandem breastfeeding positions; try different ones until you find the one that works best for you. If you have a breastfeeding café near you, go along and ask them to help you position your babies to ensure they're latching on well and you're comfortable.

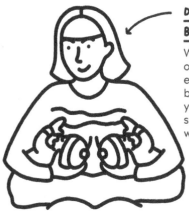

DOUBLE RUGBY BALL HOLD

With pillows or cushions on your lap, position each baby so that their bodies are tucked under your armpits and you're supporting each baby with your forearms.

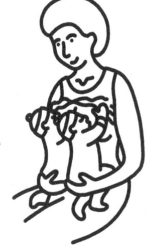

KOALA HOLD

Sit each baby on one of your thighs (it can help to prop your feet up high) and hold them in place while they feed.

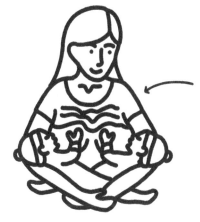

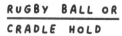

DOUBLE CRADLE HOLD

Hold each baby as if you are cradling them, allow them to latch on and then just overlap their bodies.

RUGBY BALL OR CRADLE HOLD

Place one baby in the rugby ball hold, with their body tucked under your armpit, and then position the other baby in the cradle hold.

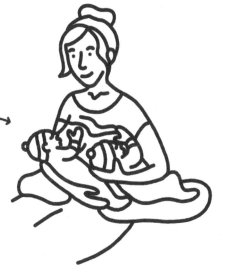

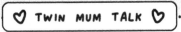

'I breastfed my twins'

NAOMI, MUM TO NON-IDENTICAL TWINS, AGED TWO,
AND A SINGLETON, AGED FOUR

I was keen to breastfeed my twins but it was difficult to find people who had breastfed twins successfully and had a positive experience – all I could find were negative stories! So while I was pregnant I prepped by doing the online breastfeeding course run by Twins Trust. As a result of the course, I felt super positive and super prepared to go into it with a, 'I'm going to do this if it's possible!' kind of attitude.

My hospital helped me harvest some breastmilk in the run up to my booked induction, which was brilliant because straight after the birth I couldn't breastfeed the babies due to bladder pain. Afterwards I was able to try tandem-feeding them. It wasn't always easy – Paloma needed light therapy for jaundice and could only come off the lamp for 20 minutes and Xanthe had low blood sugar so I could only breastfeed her every three hours so that they could test her blood-sugar levels.

Once we got the twins home, the support we had from the community midwife was amazing. She'd check the latch and answer any questions I had. After those tricky first few weeks things got much easier and I ended up feeding both twins for around 20 months. My advice to a twin mum would be just to believe that you can do it. Find the advice that you need – contact Twins Trust because they can help you, call any help lines you can and find a support network.

COMMON TWIN BREASTFEEDING QUESTIONS

I was asked these questions a lot by friends and twin mums-to-be . . .

Did you feed both babies at the same time?

I did but I know other twin mums who much preferred to feed one at a time – waking one twin to feed and then the other.

Did you feed them both at the same time even if one wasn't awake?

They were both so sleepy all of the time (which is normal for premature babies) that we had to wake them both for their feeds anyway. Later, when they were a few months old, we were in a bit of a 'nap, feed, play' routine, so we'd wake them from their nap every four hours and feed them at the same time.

What kind of breastfeeding pillow did you use?

In hospital we just used pillows and back at home, I used my pregnancy pillow, which worked fine for us but I know other twin mums who swear by the special twin-feeding pillows you can buy.

Did you switch babies to the other breast on each feed?

Yes, I tried to alternate, so I'd remember which twin was on which breast and put them on the other side next feed.

What did you do to care for your nipples with two babies breastfeeding from them?

Lots of lots of lanolin nipple cream! They weren't too bad (compared with when I breastfed my first daughter) but nipple cream is your friend.

If you bottle-feed your twins . . .

There can be a hundred reasons why you decide to – or have to – bottle-feed your twins. Some mums are much happier feeding their babies this way and some really struggle with the guilt because we so often hear, 'breast is best'.

But the simple fact is this: the most important things are that your babies are fed and that you look after your own wellbeing. So if you're finding breastfeeding twins too hard or it's affecting your mental health or just making you miserable, you don't have to do it.

And if you desperately want to breastfeed them but can't for any reason don't beat yourself up. All you can do is the best you can. You're not superwoman. Your babies will be absolutely fine and happy being fed in other ways.

Lactation Consultant Kathryn Stagg says:

'Remember, however you choose to feed and look after your babies is your business and nobody else's. You should never feel guilty about doing your best. It can be very difficult to establish breastfeeding. Also it is important to remember that if breastfeeding exclusively is not working for you, it is totally possible to do a bit of both – it does not have to be all or nothing. I am all for maximising breast milk intake for as long as possible but it can be alongside some formula if necessary. But if you decide it is not for you then it is nobody else's business. If you're struggling to breastfeed, ask for help from a breastfeeding specialist before you decide to give up. Often a few tweaks in latch make a massive difference. And in the long run, breastfeeding is super easy once you get the first couple of months out of the way.'

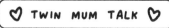

'I bottle-fed my twins'

AMY, MUM OF TEN-YEAR-OLD TWIN GIRLS,
AND AN EIGHT-YEAR-OLD SINGLETON

Tabitha was the smaller twin and needed a cup feed after birth to boost her blood sugar. I'm not sure if that led to feeding problems or if that was just her inclination, but while Georgina would gamely hold on and suck one boob while I faffed about with her sister, Tabitha would only latch on for a wee drink before losing interest. I tried her on a bottle of expressed milk and she took much more that way, so it was clear that bottle-feeding suited her better.

I moved on to expressed milk and then combi-fed them with formula but I beat myself up about it for so long (especially as my next baby, Martha, was a breeze to feed, so I breastfed her until she was eight months old).

I had been so determined to breastfeed them and I felt they were missing out on something, some kind of bonding. I think that's why I stopped breastfeeding them both – it would have felt as though Georgina was getting special treatment somehow if I kept breastfeeding her. But in truth, introducing bottles gave them a way to bond with their dad too.

Looking back, I shouldn't have felt guilty – all three of my girls have grown up happy and healthy.

HOW TO bottle-feed your twins

You might find feeding them one at a time is easier, but there are ways you can bottle-feed two hungry babies at once.

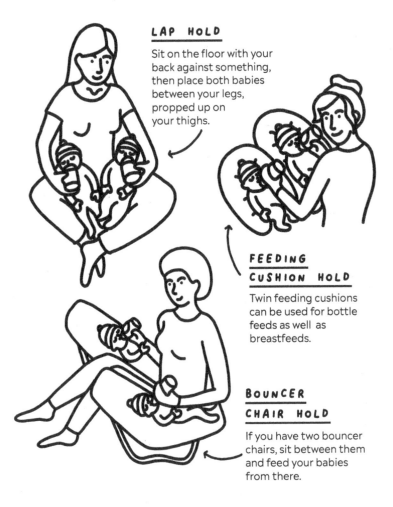

LAP HOLD

Sit on the floor with your back against something, then place both babies between your legs, propped up on your thighs.

FEEDING CUSHION HOLD

Twin feeding cushions can be used for bottle feeds as well as breastfeeds.

BOUNCER CHAIR HOLD

If you have two bouncer chairs, sit between them and feed your babies from there.

IF YOU ONLY DO 3 THINGS

1 Don't put pressure on yourself to feed your babies in a certain way – all you can do is your best in the situation you're in.

2 Keep a log of feeds for each twin to help you keep track.

3 Seek out support when you need it – look for breastfeeding cafes, lactation consultants and online feeding groups.

FOURTH TRIMESTER JOURNAL

TODAY, I AM *feeling*:

TODAY, I **NEED**:

I CAN ASK

FOR SOME **HELP**

TODAY, I AM **GRATEFUL** FOR...

FOURTH
TRIMESTER

First coined by American paediatrician, Dr Harvey Karp, the fourth trimester describes the first three months of your babies' lives. The thinking is that you should treat it as if your babies are still inside the womb - and spend the time cuddling them in a peaceful environment. It's also a concept that benefits you too - you'll likely have spent the last part of your pregnancy resting lots. If you see this 'fourth trimester' as being an extension of that same pregnancy and birth experience, and get lots of rest, it'll help your physical and mental health recovery hugely.

Chapter 12

Your physical recovery *(*and clench*)*

So you're at home getting to know your brand-new twins, dealing with everything that each day (and night) is throwing at you. On top of all of that there's the (not-so-small) matter of your physical recovery to think about. Your mental health is a big consideration right now (see page 190) but your physical health is important too. We're so good at looking after our babies when they're newborn, but in this fourth trimester period you need to look after yourself too. Rest, nourishment and doing what you can to encourage healing will all help make you stronger in these weeks.

Whether you've had a vaginal delivery or Caesarean section, chances are, there's some healing that needs to happen down below. Perhaps you've had stitches on a tear or episiotomy (when they cut the perineum to help the birth) or you could be suffering from haemorrhoids. And of course, there's the night sweats that so many of us get . . .

Lots of first-time mums are surprised when their body doesn't 'snap back' to how it was pre-pregnancy (largely, thanks to the celeb mags showing stars back in their skinny jeans a week after having a baby!) but if you consider that it took nine months for your body to grow your babies and change to accommodate

THINGS TO
ACHIEVE TODAY:

☐ feed babies
☐ rest
☐ drink lots of water
(+ MAYBE EAT A BROWNIE
OR TWO?)

them, it's not surprising that your body needs just as long (longer even) to readjust after birth. Your tummy might be 'baggy' as your uterus contracts and your organs shift back into place after pregnancy. If you've had a C-section, you might develop a bit of a 'pouch' above your scar.

The recovery from my Caesarean section was the thing that worried me most in the run up to it. I wasn't too bothered about the actual procedure – I'd had surgery before – but the recovery process was a concern. How much pain would I be in and how much of a challenge would it be to care for two small babies while I was recovering?

The surgeries I'd had before had been key hole, but this? This was major abdominal surgery. Thankfully, though, my recovery was far swifter and easier than I'd feared.

My C-section recovery
a rough timeline

Days after giving birth	What was happening/ How I felt
0 days	My lower body was still anaesthetised after the birth, so I couldn't feel a thing.
1 day	When the feeling returned to my lower body I tried to get up out of bed but couldn't manage to walk even one step. Later that day, though, I managed to shuffle - with a great deal of help - to the loo. I was taking regular painkillers and had a daily injection of a blood thinner.
2 days	I was able to shower and go to the loo, shuffling there slowly without any help. I was still in a fair amount of pain but could already see the improvement from the day before. My abdominal area was very tender and 'bloated'. I was taking regular painkillers and had a daily injection of a blood thinner.
3 days	Showering and walking to the loo became a little easier than the day before. I was taking regular painkillers and had a daily injection of a blood thinner.

4 days	Still in hospital, I managed to shuffle all the way to the tea trolley, which was up the corridor in the maternity ward.
	Every day moving felt a bit easier and less painful.
	I was taking regular painkillers and had a daily injection of a blood thinner.
5 days	We were discharged from hospital and I was able to walk up and down the hospital corridor a few times and walk to the car (my husband carried the twins in their car seats!).
	I was taking regular painkillers and had a daily injection of a blood thinner.
6 days	Back at home I was able to gently move around the house as normal. Other people lifted anything heavy for me and I was careful not to overdo it.
	I was was taking regular painkillers and had a daily injection of a blood thinner.

As the days and weeks passed, my body slowly but surely recovered. On **Day 10** I left the house for the first time since leaving the hospital and (with my husband pushing the double pram) we just slowly ambled around the block. It was enough for me at that point!

We were taking shifts through the night (see more on page 202) and when I woke to feed the babies I'd find myself drenched in sweat. There would be no time to shower, so I'd change into dry pyjamas and head downstairs. While night sweats aren't pleasant, they're totally normal and a result of your hormone levels adjusting and your body getting rid of lots of excess fluid.

If you're recovering from a C-section . . .

* You may be encouraged to get out of bed and move around as soon as you can in hospital.

* Go slowly and don't expect too much of your body. There are lots of layers of tissue which need to heal in your body.

* Embrace the giant pants! A nice high waistband that sits above your scar and 100 per cent cotton are good, so they're a nice breathable fabric.

* You might have some vaginal bleeding (make those giant pants dark in colour!) so stock up on sanitary pads.

* Gently clean and pat dry your wound every day – and keep an eye out for any signs of infection.

* You're discouraged from lifting anything heavier than your baby for six weeks and you won't be able to drive, exercise or have sex for that period too (but it might be even longer until you feel like doing any of those things).

VAGINAL BLEEDING

Vaginal bleeding happens after the birth, regardless of whether it was a vaginal or Caesarean delivery – you might need heavy duty sanitary pads (it's not advisable to use tampons for six weeks) and big dark-coloured cotton pants for comfort.

If you're recovering from a vaginal birth . . .

❋ You might have stitches from a tear or episiotomy (cut to the perineum) and if so, bathe them in warm water (no bubble bath) every day and pat dry.

❋ The first time you go to the loo can be daunting – your vagina and vulva can feel tender and swollen and sometimes urinating can sting. You might also feel nervous about that first postnatal poo! It can help to support the perineum by gently placing a wad of loo roll or a pad against it while you try to relax your bowels. It's important not to get constipated so drink lots of water and eat fresh fruit and veg.

The six-week check up

Six weeks after having your twins you should have a check-up with you GP to make sure you're feeling OK and recovering properly. Your babies might also be checked over at the same time or you might have separate appointments for each of you.

Your GP will usually take your blood pressure, ask about vaginal discharge and bleeding, check your Caesarean scar if you have one, ask you about your mental health and ask you what contraception you're using (at this point, you're very welcome to simply point to the two babies next to you and smile. 'I had twins six weeks ago,' I wanted to say, when asked this. 'Do you think I'm having sex?'). Your GP might also weigh you and chat to you about healthy eating.

3 things that you need to know about your postnatal recovery

Anya Hayes (@mothers.wellness.toolkit), Pilates instructor and author specialising in pre- and postnatal vitality and self-compassion

1 Even though you've been 'signed off' at your six-week check, your body is still healing

The six-week postnatal check typically marks the formal end of maternity care in England. But at six weeks your body is far from 'back to normal' – you're not yet fully healed and you are still postnatal forever. Six weeks leaves just enough time for the first stage of soft tissue to heal. It can take several months for the abdominal and pelvic muscles to recover fully, for your connective tissue to completely firm up and organs to have reassembled themselves into the space your babies have left. This process will take longer if you're breastfeeding because of the ongoing hormonal fluctuation in your body.

2 The six-week postnatal check only skims the surface

You may be surprised by how cursory your six-week check is – often mums report now that it's about the baby, with possibly a question about contraception, which, let's face it, may feel like the least relevant issue right now. GPs have a lot to cover on the health of mum and babies in a very short appointment, and with twins particularly you may feel that your needs are entirely squeezed out. Be ready to mention anything which doesn't seem quite right, and don't assume that not being asked about something means it's a normal after-effect of childbirth. Make sure you tell your GP if you're struggling with incontinence or flatulence, if sex is painful or if you have the sensation of something heavy in your vagina as this can be a symptom of prolapse. Any of these things can indicate the need for further follow-up or onward referral. In a nutshell, all women should really see a physio post birth, but particularly if you've carried twins or multiples. But currently that's not in the standard pathway of care, so you may need to proactively seek it as a treatment option for you.

3 You need to strengthen your core first and foremost

Pregnancy hinders the ability of your core to work effectively, as there were two living babies affecting (and sabotaging!) the connections you normally require to be strong and functional. Your core is your body's stability system: the diaphragm at the top, the pelvic floor at the bottom, the transverse abdominis (TVA) at the front and the multifidus at the back. The core doesn't automatically return to a functional way of working immediately after birth or, magically, when you reach six weeks postpartum.

We need to re-educate your postnatal core to work together as a team, whether you gave birth vaginally or via C-section. Let's take the TVA muscle as an example. This is the deepest of your four abdominal muscles and has attachments to your pelvic floor. As your bump grows, your TVA stretches: and with two babies, you can imagine this stretching is even more than with a single pregnancy. It's placed in this lengthened position for months and, as a result, becomes weakened. Juggling two newborn babies is uniquely stressful on body and mind and you need to allow some time for your body to rebuild its strength by accepting that you need some attention too. Reject the 'bounceback' in favour of finding your way home to a body you feel safe and comfortable in.

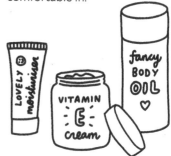

Exercises that are <u>safe</u> to do and will <u>help</u> you recover

<u>Pelvic-floor exercises</u>

Pelvic-floor exercises, with deep conscious breathing, promote healing and help you to regain the strength of the pelvic floor. Start your pelvic floor exercises as soon as possible, however your babies were delivered. Download the NHS Squeezy app and follow its reminders. And yes, this is just as important after a Caesarean birth. The sooner the better, so (as long as any catheter has been removed) you can begin even while your anaesthetic is wearing off, to help with blood supply and circulation. Pelvic floor exercises are not 'something else to do' – like breathing exercises, it's more supercharging something you are already doing, building the awareness into your every day habits. That is what will make the overall difference to your pelvic floor health.

How to do pelvic floor exercises . . .

To do your pelvic floor exercises correctly, draw up your back passage as if trying to stop breaking wind, then travel that engagement forward and up. Try not to hold your breath while finding your pelvic floor; focus on timing the squeeze-and-lift manoeuvre with an out-breath, and then allow the entire pelvic floor to relax on the inhale. Do a few repetitions slowly and intentionally three times every day.

PELVIC FLOOR EXERCISE REWARD CHART

Day	Done	Reward
MONDAY	☐	BROWNIE WITH YOUR MORNING CUPPA
TUESDAY	☐	BUBBLE BATH
WEDNESDAY	☐	EXTRA EPISODE OF GILMORE GIRLS
THURSDAY	☐	FOOT RUB
FRIDAY	☐	HALF AN HOUR TO SIT IN SILENCE

Pilates

Pilates is uniquely appropriate for post-birth recovery, focusing on pelvic floor and abdominal function, on posture awareness and releasing tension built up every day.

The one exercise I do every single day without fail is Spine Curls.

* *Lie on your back, with knees bent, feet flat on the floor.*

* *Soften and lengthen your body into the floor.*

* *Take a few slow deep breaths. On an out breath, press your feet lightly into the floor and tilt your pelvis in towards you to begin to peel your spine up from the floor, bone by bone, like a string of pearls. Roll up gently to around the centre of your shoulder blades. Take a deep breath in there, holding your buttocks firm to lift the weight of your pelvis, then slowly roll the spine down, bone by bone. Imagine it's like a bicycle chain, evenly rolling.*

* *Repeat this five to 10 times, becoming more aware of your body's sensation and strength with each one.*

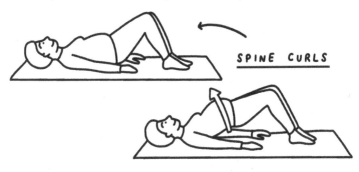

SPINE CURLS

If you go to a Pilates class, check that they're qualified in postnatal exercise prescription, regardless of the fact that you've had the 'sign-off' at your postnatal check.

What to expect from a pelvic health physio check up

Helen Keeble (@helenkeeblephysio),
clinical specialist physio in pelvic health

The best time to go for a pelvic health physio check-up is eight weeks after birth, but it's never too late. Eight weeks is ideal because then everything has shrunk back down again and we know exactly what we're working with.

At the appointment we check how your pelvic-floor muscles are recovering because even if you had a C-section your pelvic floor gets weakened during pregnancy. So we'll check what the strength of your muscles is, check your technique is still working well, check what your endurance is, and then we will make an exercise programme for you.

We can also check for prolapse and if you had an episiotomy or tear, then we can check that as well and just make sure that that's all OK. I often get women worrying about vaginal scars before they have sex again. So it can be really reassuring for them to have them checked.

Then we will be checking the lower back and the pelvis, to make sure that they're in good alignment and moving really well. We'll also be checking their tummy for a diastasis recti.

We really focus in on the core – so exactly where the babies were growing and the impact that had on your body. Because unfortunately, we don't all just bounce back, you know, it does kind of take a bit of work. It's not hard work though! It's normally just a few key things. It really helps your body recover in the best way – you're future proofing things for having other babies or, if you're not having any more babies, for the menopause.

FIVE QUICK SNACK IDEAS THAT WILL NOURISH YOUR POSTNATAL BODY

It can often feel hard to eat well when you're looking after newborn twins so being prepared with some healthy, nourishing snacks can really help. Eating little and often can be a great way to keep your blood-sugar levels stable and hunger pangs at bay!

1. **Wholemeal pitta bread dipped into hummus**
   Wholemeal bread and whole grains are great for getting your bowels regular in the fourth trimester.

2. **Lactation cookies**
   If you're breastfeeding, buy (or ask a friend to make – recipe opposite) some lactation cookies. They contain lots of vitamins and minerals and they're believed to help boost your milk supply.

3. **A few squares of dark chocolate**
   Packed with minerals that your body needs, it's a great excuse to enjoy some chocolate.

4. **Mashed avocado on wholegrain toast**
   Add a poached egg for some extra protein.

5. **Celery dipped in peanut butter**
   This will give you a great energy boost and celery is a diuretic so it can help with all that excess fluid you might have in the early days post-birth.

Quick & Easy No-Bake Lactation Bites

Meg Routhorn from Mothers Love Cookies (@motherslovecookies)

The key ingredients in this recipe are oats, flaxseed and brewer's yeast – which are all believed to boost milk supply and give you a hit of energy.

INGREDIENTS

200g oats
60g milled flaxseed
30g brewer's yeast
  powder
300g peanut butter *
180g honey **
1 teaspoon vanilla extract
1 teaspoon ground
  cinnamon (*optional*)
100g chocolate chips
  (*optional*)
100g dried fruit or nuts
  (*optional*)

*any nut or seed butter will work (almond butter, cashew butter, sunflower seed butter, etc.)

**replace honey with maple syrup or agave syrup to make recipe vegan-friendly

METHOD

1 Add oats, flaxseed, brewer's yeast, peanut butter, honey, vanilla and cinnamon to a bowl or mixer fitted with a paddle attachment.

2 Mix until well combined.

3 Stir in chocolate and/or dried fruit and nuts (if using).

4 Roll mixture into small balls (approximately 1 tablespoon each, about 3 cm in diameter) and place on a parchment paper lined baking tray or press the entire mixture into a parchment paper lined 20 x 20cm baking tin.

5 Refrigerate for 30 minutes or until set.

6 Transfer bites to an airtight container. They will keep for up to a week in the refrigerator or freeze for up to three months.

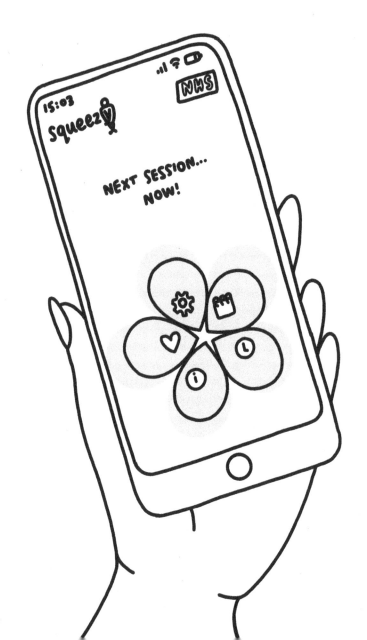

IF YOU ONLY DO 3 THINGS

1 Download the Squeezy app and start doing pelvic-floor exercises as soon as possible.

2 Ask your GP to refer you for a physiotherapy appointment.

3 Snack on nourishing food that will help your physical and emotional recovery.

Chapter 13

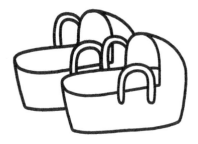

The first few weeks at home with twins

Arriving home from the hospital with our small newborn twins created a total mixed bag of emotions inside me. It was such a relief to be getting back to our own surroundings and we were desperate to spend time with our eldest daughter after five days in hospital away from her. But I was also nervous. In hospital, we'd had help from midwives at the touch of a button, but at home we'd have to work stuff out for ourselves or turn to Dr Google for advice.

We were discharged at 8pm – around 12 hours after we'd been told we could go home.

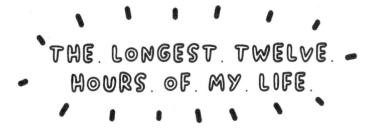

THE. LONGEST. TWELVE. HOURS. OF. MY. LIFE.

We assumed we'd be gone by lunchtime but every time we asked, a midwife told us they were still trying to get our discharge papers signed. We packed our bags and waited. And waited. When the papers finally came, I practically skipped out of the ward.

We were taking our babies home!

We knew our eight-year-old was waiting up past her bedtime to see us all and when we walked through the door it was such a lovely moment. Hugs and smiles all around. Then we all just sat on the sofa, with the babies sleeping in their car seats, looking at them in wonder.

Once we'd tucked our eldest into bed, we weirdly felt at a slightly loose end. Both babies were asleep in their cot and we sat next to them wondering what to do! We'd been in such a good rhythm and routine in the hospital; we were going to have to – I guess – create a new routine at home.

Over the next few days we carried on feeding the twins every three hours – breastfeed, formula, expressed milk – and I would then express for the next feed. Sometimes, after all of that, I only had an hour before it was time for the next feed, which at times felt relentless. But I tried to use that short amount of time to rest – doing skin to skin with the babies or watching something trashy on Netflix.

We decided not to have lots of visitors in those first few weeks at home. At the hospital, our eldest and my mum (who was staying at ours and looking after her) had come to visit but nobody else. Once we were home, my husband's mum and dad came to meet their new granddaughters, but other than that, we didn't have anyone else visit. It was really important to me that we had a quiet spell to get to know the babies, to get ourselves into some kind of routine and, crucially, to not feel like we had to tidy the house, make cups of tea and be 'hosts' to anyone, no matter how dear a friend they were. Back when we'd had our first daughter, we had loads of people over to visit from the off. I was worrying about having nice biscuits in and offering to make hot drinks because – well, that's what you do, isn't it? No. When you've just had a baby (or two!) it's totally fine to either put people off from coming over (you don't have to be rude, you can just say you're having a few weeks of quiet before inviting people over) or if you do have people over, don't move from that sofa!

'You know where the kettle is!' is a really good phrase to chuck at anyone who comes over. It'll soon jog them into help mode and, if they're a really good friend, they'll give the kitchen a quick wipe down and hang up some laundry while they're waiting for the kettle to boil!

We did, of course, have midwives and health visitors pop round – they were always a friendly face and thankfully full of encouraging words. They'd weigh the babies, chat about how we were getting on with feeds and we could ask any questions we had. I got into a habit of scribbling down any questions ready to ask them and we were still making a note of every feed (this actually became our eldest's job whenever she was around . . . 'So, you did 20 minutes BF? And 5ml EBF? And 5ml formula?' she'd ask before scribbling it down in the notebook).

It was a strange old time though. If this was the 1990s, I'd be sharing a handwritten diary entry with you, but it's the 2020s, so this is what I wrote on Instagram a few days after we'd come home from hospital:

I admit it – I'd totally forgotten what this hazy sleep-deprived fog that you experience when you have a newborn baby (or two) was like. I'm wandering around in a slightly confused state, unsure what day it is. I've got leaky boobs, the night sweats and a C-section scar that I can't even see yet because I've still got a big squishy bump. All the glamour here, folks! It's all good though & we have totally pulled up the drawbridge – we've had no visitors,

I haven't left the house since we got back from hospital and my days/nights just revolve around feeding, cuddling and resting.

The Newborn Fog is a definite, real thing. And like I said on social media, I'd totally forgotten about it until it hit me again. It's one of those all-consuming experiences that you can't even fathom until it's happened to you. The combination of hormones, sleep-deprivation and getting your head around the enormity of being responsible for these new, tiny humans throws you into a hazy existence where you're really not sure what day it is.

It's pretty understandable when you think about the sheer enormity of what your body has just been through and everything that's involved with caring for two newborns.

I spent a good few weeks in the Newborn Fog. When midwives and health visitors came over to do the standard check-ups, even the simplest of questions would leave me stumped. 'Which baby is this?' she'd ask as I handed her one to weigh. Me: 'Ermmm . . .'

I'd look out of the window of my living room and the outside world seemed like an alternate universe. People were going about their everyday business – going to work, popping to the shops, walking dogs – yet here I was in this bizarre existence where my main focus was keeping two small babies alive, my day was divided up into three-hourly feeding segments, and it was all happening in ever so slightly slow motion thanks to the lack of sleep I was getting.

The Newborn Fog gradually started to lift, and after a few months my head started to clear. Things felt a bit more normal and each day was a bit less like wading through treacle, in slow motion.

HOW TO survive the first few weeks at home

Mars Lord (@_marslord), doula and twin mum

GET YOUR POSTNATAL PLAN IN PLACE WHILE YOU'RE PREGNANT

It's a bit like getting married, we plan the wedding but we forget what happens afterwards. Think about who's going to be there for you and what does that support look like?

THINK ABOUT WHO WOULD BE USEFUL TO HAVE AROUND YOU IN THOSE EARLY DAYS

It can be great to have family and friends come over to help, but who are the people that will come and be useful, and who are the ones that will come and cause you more work and stress? What type of family do you have? Are you a 'doors open, everybody in' kind of family? Or are you very private and closed and so you don't want people coming in and out of your house?

PREP YOUR PARTNER, OR A CLOSE FAMILY MEMBER, TO BE YOUR GATEKEEPER

The best support you can have is the person who's there, supporting you at home. Whether it's your partner or a family member, they're the one who lets people in and out of that door. One of my best memories of when I had my twins was when I had a couple of friends that arrived at my front door and I remember thinking, 'Oh, f*** off.' I really had no time for any more people to come and visit, but they said, 'We've not come see you and we're not interested in the babies.' I looked down and they were both carrying buckets and yellow gloves. I heard them singing in my bathroom as they cleaned it from top to bottom. Then I heard them singing in the kitchen as they were cleaning. And then they

put their heads around the door and said, 'You might need to turn the oven off in about 45 minutes! There's a lasagne in there' and they left. Just brilliant. Absolute queens. But your partner is your first gatekeeper. Your partner is the one who will let people in and kick people out.

HOW YOU'RE FEELING WHEN YOU GET HOME FROM HOSPITAL CAN DEPEND ON HOW LONG YOU WERE IN FOR

If you've managed to be discharged within a day or so, then you're more likely to hit the ground running and do OK, but it's normal to still feel overwhelmed. It's normal to have a real sense of 'Well, what do we do now?' If you've been in hospital for a few days – maybe you've had a Caesarean section, maybe because it's twins the hospital have kept you there until they're happy with the way the babies are feeding – then you might become that little bit institutionalised. You could be used to turning around to call for someone to help.

WHEN YOU'RE PREGNANT, ASK FRIENDS TO ORGANISE A MEAL TRAIN

When I had my twins, the church that I used to go to planned a meal train – each person had a day assigned to them and they'd bring me a home-cooked meal. You'll find that in the different faith groups – mosques, synagogues, churches and the like – there are always people who will do that. So think about who's going to be your meal train? Because it's hard getting food when you have one baby. So when you have two babies, your hands are very rarely empty. Or you might like to prepare to fill your freezer in the run up to the birth.

SUPPORT NETWORK

CONSIDER HIRING A POSTNATAL DOULA (SEE PAGE 183)

Postnatal doulas come in for a set number of hours through the day and that might allow you space to have a bath or just not hold a baby for ten minutes or cook a meal, or just have a break. Of course, not everyone can afford a doula – or a night nanny, which seems popular with twin families – so if that's the case, think about what support you can get from your local children's centre. A great resource is Homestart (homestart.org.uk) – a home help service with volunteers who'll come out to help you. There might be a local college with people studying to be nursery nurses who could help you.

PREPARE YOURSELF FOR THE RELENTLESSNESS OF IT ALL

Now, relentless doesn't mean awful, it just means it keeps going. No one prepares us for this when we have twins. We somehow have this impression that we will have these blocks of time when we're doing nothing, when we're sitting back and resting. But I think if we were prepared for the relentlessness, it would be so much easier. But what happens is people don't talk about that, we get there, we're in the middle of it and suddenly, we panic. It doesn't have to be that way. And it doesn't last forever!

A word on doulas

Lots of twin mums and experts recommend postnatal doulas for twin mums, but what are they? Doulas provide emotional and practical support for a family. Usually booked for a certain number of hours or days each week, they might come to your home and help with domestic tasks, look after the babies while you nap, help look after siblings or cook meals for you.

I'll be honest with you – I used to think they were just for incredibly wealthy people. Imagine having the money to pay for someone to come, help you around the house and look after you and your babies! But I've since discovered that they're a lot more accessible than I'd thought. I know some new mums who have booked one for just a few hours each week, and it's been enough to make a difference to how they're coping.

There are also ways that people on lower incomes can access doula help. Doula UK have an access fund which you can apply for, and it allows new mums who are on low incomes to access doula support free of charge. Eligibility criteria is on the Doulas UK website.

There's also an organisation called Neighbourhood Doulas – if you are a vulnerable parent, under 25 or you have no partner, they have some funding so that they can support you for free over a certain period of time.

3 EASY MEALS

THAT I CAN COOK *ahead* OF TIME/
ASK FRIENDS TO DROP OVER...

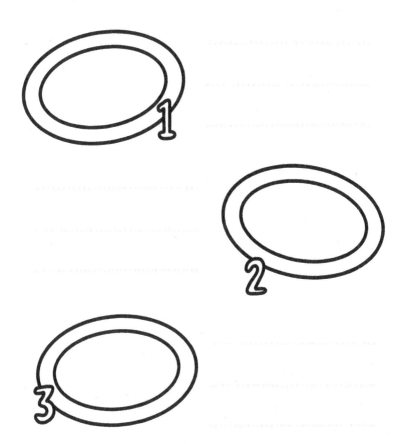

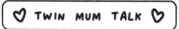

'Batch cooking one-pot meals was a sanity saver for me'

SARAH, MUM TO SEVEN-YEAR-OLD NON-IDENTICAL TWINS

I didn't exactly have my planned twin birth. I ended up having George with forceps and then an emergency C-section for Harriet 20 minutes later. It was physically very hard but on the plus side, they were both big and well enough to not be in special care, which was a total relief.

We had no family help nearby, so after taking advice from a couple of friends who had had twins recently, I knew we had to be organised when they arrived. Something that helped hugely was batch cooking. When we did our NCT course, one of the (only?!) useful things (apart from my new friends) was when the course leader asked us to really pin-point what was our own pressure point. What was one thing we needed to function, or what would make us feel out of control if we didn't have them. For some people it was sleep, or time alone or a tidy house, but for me I knew it was home-cooked food. I knew that if we lived in food chaos, I'd feel grim. So I set about tackling that point in advance of the babies arriving. I prepared and froze (I kid you not) hundreds of portions of meals. Nothing fancy, just casseroles and one-pot meals. Our freezer was bursting. When we were in the dark days of sleepless nights and lonely days of constant feeding, crying and mess, those meals gave me so much comfort. I think really considering your own pressure point before and tackling in advance is a brilliant tactic and one which really helped me.

'I found the first few weeks at home with my twins totally overwhelming'

KIRSTY, MUM TO TEN-YEAR-OLD BOY/GIRL TWINS

I arrived home from the hospital with two very small babies and feeling terrified. Their arrival into the world wasn't at all what I'd expected and planned for. During my pregnancy, I'd developed obstetric cholestasis, which meant my liver started to pack up and I was covered in hives, so the twins had to be delivered by emergency C-section at 36 weeks. My girl twin, Artemis, had jaundice and was put in an incubator, but the incubator malfunctioned and she overheated and had to be resuscitated. It was all pretty traumatic. I was also dealing with huge patches of my skin reddening and falling off because of the obstetric cholestasis. And the babies had to be cup-fed, because they had no sucking reflex. I wasn't even able to try to breastfeed them because I was on steroids to sort out my liver and skin – I found this really hard to come to terms with.

So because of all of that, when I got home with the twins, I wasn't in a great place and I found everything overwhelming. I vividly remember thinking that it was all down to me now and that if the hospital couldn't even get things right, I had to do it all myself to protect the twins.

I felt the weight of the world on me and I just freaked out. I couldn't sleep, I couldn't eat and I wouldn't talk about it with anyone. The slightest thing would overwhelm me – one day, my niece-in-law came to see the twins and when she left, she told me she was off to meet her mum and go and see a movie. I sobbed for hours, so convinced was I that I would never, ever be able to do anything like that myself again. I also felt incredibly guilty because we'd had IVF to have the twins, so I knew we were incredibly lucky to even have them.

My close friends had been on this journey with me, too, but having always been open to discussing difficult things with them, I suddenly felt that I was letting the side down if I told them how completely desperate I felt. Luckily for me, three weeks in, a friend, who lived close by, refused to accept my excuses as to why she couldn't come to visit and she turned up one day to find me exhausted and tearful with two fractious babies. She frogmarched me down to the doctors where fortunately, the GP I spoke to understood and provided a safe space for me to explore why I was feeling the way I was, and what options my were.

After lots of talking, I realised I needed to accept help when it was offered (I've never been good at that). We made the decision to blow my maternity pay on getting a night nanny, twice a week, from 7pm to 7am. We're so lucky that we were in a position where we could afford to do this, but it really did save me. Previously, I'd been averaging around three hours of sleep each night but knowing that twice a week I had someone to hand the twins over to, which would allow me to sleep, helped me to see things in a more realistic light. I appreciated that life would forever be different but it would not always be this intense emotional roller coaster. Gradually, I began to feel better.

If I could give one piece of advice to someone who is finding the first few weeks at home overwhelming it would be this: there isn't just one solution to handling twins but take help when it is offered, in whatever form it's offered. If it's not offered, actively seek it; it makes all the difference.

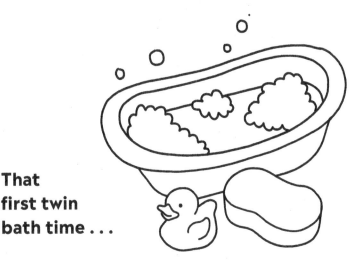

That first twin bath time . . .

One of the things that many twin mums worry about is bathing twins. We (still to this day!) only bathe ours when we are both around to help, but it's totally possible to do it on your own. It doesn't have to be an overwhelming task, and it's one of those things that the more you do it, the easier it will feel. Here's some information about bathing twins that I hope will be useful:

* You don't have to bathe them every day.

* You can bathe them at any time of the day – it doesn't have to be just before bed.

* Bathe them separately – you can have one on a towel or mat, on the floor while you bathe the other.

* If you use a baby bath, you can place it on a higher surface to make it easier to do.

* Have everything you need to hand before you start – baby wash, towels, nappies and fresh babygrows.

* Have soothing music of your choice playing (this is as much for you, as it is for the babies).

IF YOU ONLY DO 3 THINGS

1 Plan what your support system will look like when the babies arrive. Write it down and chat to the people involved about what you'll need from them.

2 Think about meals - do you want to batch cook and freeze? Ask friends to create a meal train? Sign up to a (pricey but handy) meal kit service?

3 Be ready for the relentlessness of these early days. It will get easier.

Chapter 14

Your postnatal mental health
(How are you feeling?)

We're getting so much better at talking about mental health, aren't we? When you really stop to think about it, it should be no different to talking about our physical health. Chatting about feeling low or anxious today should be as normal as mentioning you've been getting headaches or you've got a sore back. But there's still a stigma attached to mental health issues – a stigma that's thankfully lessening as we talk about it more, and as we realise that pretty much all of us at some point in our life will be affected by some kind of mental-health issue.

During my twin pregnancy, one of the main things I was worried about was my mental health in the postnatal period.
I had really struggled when my first daughter was a baby. Back then, getting through each day felt like a huge challenge. Sitting in a coffee shop, I'd look around me and see all of these mums with their babies, appearing to be totally nailing the motherhood thing. They looked bright-eyed and happy, they coped when their baby cried, they looked chilled out, like they were taking everything in their stride. In contrast, I felt like sobbing pretty much all the time and it felt so hard. My baby crying in the

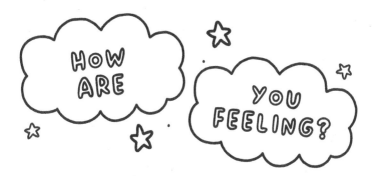

supermarket would send me into a panic and if I realised mid-nappy change that I'd come out of the house without any baby wipes, I'd burst into tears and feel useless.

I struggled being at home on my own with my baby after being so used to busying about every day. But getting out with her to a baby class or to meet a friend for coffee just seemed so difficult too.

Even when we'd put her to bed in the evening I'd find myself unable to relax. We'd put a film on but I'd sit there a ball of anxiety, wondering if the TV volume was too high and would wake her up.

At the time, I had no idea that I was suffering from postnatal depression. I'd heard of it, of course, but it didn't click that this was the problem. I thought that motherhood was just really hard and while most people managed to cope fine, I was crumbling under the weight of my new role.

It was when my daughter was 18 months old that the penny dropped. I was reading a blog post written by a mum with postnatal depression. 'I wonder . . . is that what I've had?' I asked myself. I was largely better by then, so told myself there wasn't much point in getting any professional help, but there was also a part of me that thought: 'What if I go to see the GP and she tells me that it wasn't postnatal depression?' The idea of a health professional confirming my worst fear – that *I'm just pretty rubbish at motherhood* – was too much to bear. I realise now that just the fact that I was having these ludicrous thoughts probably indicates that I wasn't 100 per cent well and should have sought help.

So during my twin pregnancy I was incredibly worried that history would repeat itself. But I was determined to handle it differently if it did. 'At the first sign that I'm not feeling OK, I'm going straight to the GP,' I told my husband.

Thankfully, when the twins arrived, history didn't repeat itself. Partly, I think, because I was so much more in tune with my mental health than I used to be. I've become much better at listening to how I'm feeling, recognising signs that I need to rest or ask for help. But also, I suspect, because I ensured that I had sufficient support in those first few weeks and months of twin motherhood. I knew how hard having one baby had been, so there was no way I was going to try to do this alone. I asked for help and I accepted any help that was offered. When my mum – who stayed with us for the first couple of weeks – ushered me off to bed for an hour I didn't put up a fight. I knew that in order to be the best mum I could to my three children I had to look after myself.

When I'd had my first daughter, I was desperate to, 'get back to normal life'. I put pressure on myself to get out and about, because that's what you do, isn't it? Popping to the shops, meeting my antenatal friends for coffee, going to a baby class, visiting my colleagues in the office to show off the new baby – I'd love to go back in time and say to myself: 'STOP. Just stop. You don't have to be doing all of this. It's fine if you want to sit around in your pyjamas all day drinking tea and watching daytime telly while you cuddle your baby.' I mean, there aren't many times in life when you can hang out – guilt-free – with Phillip Schofield and Holly Willoughby every morning, but this, without a doubt, is one of them.

The baby blues

The day after we got home from hospital, the community midwife came to visit us. 'How have you been feeling?' she asked me, kindly. 'It's very normal, around day four or five to feel tearful and low, and it's caused by your breastmilk coming in.' It was so brilliant to be asked about this, but I was able to assure her that I was feeling fine. 'I've actually been feeling OK!' I said brightly.

Cut to that evening and I was sitting with my husband watching *Strictly Come Dancing*. I suddenly felt totally overwhelmed by emotions and had tears streaming down my face. 'What's wrong?' my husband asked, clearly concerned by what was happening. 'I don't know!' I replied, sobbing. 'Nothing! Everything!'

Then I remembered what the midwife had said that morning. I knew that if I could get my body to produce the hormone oxytocin it would help, so I got the babies – who'd been happily sleeping next to me – and did skin to skin with them. I just sat there, still watching Strictly, but with them lying on my skin, all of us wrapped up together in a blanket. And before long, I felt so much better. It was like magic.

This temporary feeling of sadness is caused by hormone and chemical changes going on in the body post-birth. It's often called the baby blues – which if you ask me is a bit of a rubbish cutesy name for something that can make you feel low, anxious, tearful and unsettled for a few days, at least.

The good news is that the baby blues is not postnatal depression. Sitting there sobbing in front of *Strictly*, I knew from previous experience that it was just a temporary state, so I didn't panic about descending into depression.

How do I <u>know</u> if I have postnatal depression?

Twin mums are more likely to suffer from PND than other mums. This is because of increased stressful life events – hospitalisation and medicalisation around pregnancy and birth, caring for two babies, greater sleep deprivation, greater potential for social isolation, higher financial costs and more.

If you find your mood is persistently low, you're feeling anxious, or if you are experiencing any type of distress that is impacting on your day-to-day functioning then it's worth speaking to a healthcare professional. It can sometimes – as I demonstrated when I had my first daughter – be difficult to recognise that you're experiencing postnatal depression. It can develop gradually, and when you're already very sleep-deprived and on this huge learning curve, looking after two brand new babies, it can be hard to know whether it's PND or not. So even if you are unsure it's worth speaking to your GP who can chat things through with you and refer you to a perinatal mental-health service.

What <u>exactly</u> are my hormones doing right now?

Your hormones change massively when you're pregnant, and once you've given birth they adjust again, which can have a big effect on how you're feeling. 'The levels of hormones in our bodies during pregnancy are crazy,' says women's health physiotherapist Helen Keeble. 'Our progesterone is up to 600 per cent of what it is at normal times and our oestrogen is more – during one pregnancy – than it will ever be during that whole lifetime, if you add it all up.' When you consider that your body stops producing progesterone as soon as you deliver the placenta(s) and your oestrogen levels will drop more than a hundred fold in the first three days after you've given birth, it's hardly surprising that it can have a massive effect on how we feel postpartum.

THINGS THAT I
CAN'T CONTROL

- WHAT MY *hormones* ARE DOING
- HOW *tiredness* IS AFFECTING ME

....
....
(FILL IN YOUR OWN)

THINGS THAT I
CAN CONTROL

- THE *boundaries* I SET
- THE *expectations* I HAVE OF *myself*
- THE *help* I *ask* FOR
- MY *breathing*

....
....
(FILL IN YOUR OWN)

<u>HOW TO</u> look after your mental health in the fourth trimester

Dr Emma Hepburn (@thepsychologymum), clinical psychologist

1 Allow yourself to rest and recover from giving birth
Try not to put pressure on yourself to get back to your 'pre-babies life'. See this as the fourth trimester and understand what to expect during this period.

2 Manage your own expectations about what you will be doing post-birth
Surviving and helping your babies thrive as much as you can are the most realistic expectations you can have.

3 Allow some flexibility in your standards
Does it really matter if the house is messy or you decide to stay in your pyjamas all day? We just don't have capacity to do everything and at this time your and your babies' needs are the most important things there are.

4 Plan help if possible
Arrange for people to support you, particularly at vulnerable points, for example your partner's return to work.

5 Plan in small pockets of enjoyment (See page 200)

6 Remember to breathe when stress is high!
So simple, but so powerful – it engages your parasympathetic system, which is your body's soothing response, and can keep your stress in check and calm you down, just that little bit, at times of high stress (see page 106 for breathing techniques).

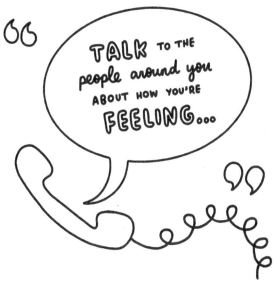

TALK TO THE *people around you* ABOUT HOW YOU'RE **FEELING...**

7 **If you're even slightly worried about your mental health, speak to your GP**

It is worth speaking to your GP or health visitor even if you are unsure as they will be able to assess you and help answer any questions you have. If you are feeling bad or distressed, it is always worth speaking to someone to help understand what is going on and work out the best way forward for you.

8 **Remember, there's nothing wrong with you if you need help**

The stigma around mental health, and what this means about you as a mother, still runs through society's veins. People can be afraid to speak up as they think it means they're not a good mother. Some even fear that their children might be taken away from them. Motherhood can be portrayed as this magical and wonderful time, which can make you feel like there is something wrong with you if you are finding it difficult.

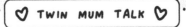

♡ TWIN MUM TALK ♡

'I suffered from postnatal depression after having twins'

HANNAH, MUM TO SIX-YEAR-OLD TWINS

The boys were born six weeks early and they were in SCBU for three weeks. During this time we were in a bit of a bubble. When we got home with them, I had a gradual descent into postnatal depression. I felt overwhelmed looking after two babies, one of whom was a bad sleeper, and both were difficult to feed thanks to reflux. Once things settled down and we got into a routine of sorts, I realised I still felt overwhelmed, isolated and a bit disengaged for the whole experience. My husband came home on numerous occasions to find me crying.

My initial health visitor was not very supportive and dismissed my concerns by saying, 'Well, you've got two babies! You're bound to be overwhelmed!' I wasn't offered any extra support. I spent a lot of time either in the house with the boys alone or taking them for long walks on my own. Due to where we lived at the time, we were rather isolated and the lack of visitors only made me feel worse.

It wasn't until they were six months old that I realised it might be postnatal depression. I saw a string of different health visitors who all convinced me I was fine and it would get easier. It took its toll on my relationship with my husband – he did his best to support me, give me breaks and allow me to be sad, angry, express myself but it was hard.

I eventually got a PND and PNA – postnatal anxiety – diagnosis but it took a long time and a lot of persistence from me. The GP prescribed me antidepressants but they didn't really help me and I didn't like the side effects so I came off them after a few months.

One thing which has had a big positive impact on my mental health is taking up running almost a year ago. It has been amazing and I really think this is what has helped me turn the corner. I've also joined a few twin groups on social media that I've found helpful and supportive and as time has gone on, I've found my 'people' on Instagram.

If you suspect you're suffering from postnatal depression, speak to someone, whether it is a friend, medical professional or an online mum group. If feel you need help push for it! You are not alone, there is support and help for you. It is hard, but you'll get through it and your feelings are valid.

If you do need some help

Treatment might include psychological interventions, such as CBT or medication (a doctor can recommend what medicine can be taken while breastfeeding). 'Many people are also able to use self-help with their PND,' says Dr Emma Hepburn, 'which can help them understand what is going on and ways to help. This can be through either (or a combination of) evidence-based online resources (such as online CBT, which is available free), exercise, speaking things through with trusted people, trouble-shooting stressors, accessing help (for example, offers of childcare) which can enable you to sleep or give you some time to yourself, breaking avoidance patterns and engaging in valued activities. This is not an exclusive list, and while some people may be able to do things to help themselves, this is not always possible, and there is no shame in requiring additional input from professionals.'

<u>HOW TO</u> find pockets of enjoyment

Treating yourself to small everyday pleasures can provide little pockets of positive effects that guide you through an overwhelming time.

1 **Listen to podcasts while you're feeding**.
Fearne Cotton's *Happy Place* might lift your mood, The Scummy Mummies could give you a laugh or if you're keen to stay in touch with the real world BBC *Woman's Hour* is a good one.

2 **Audiobooks are another great option**
Choose a nice gentle read like a Marian Keyes or JoJo Moyes novel.

3 **Schedule in an hour when your partner is on duty with the twins and you take yourself off for a soak in the bath.**
(Refrain from having a bath until three days after giving birth if you've had stitches but after that, bath or shower every day and gently pat the area dry with a towel.)

IF YOU ONLY DO 3 THINGS

1 Don't worry if you get a wave of the baby blues. It will pass.

2 Tell your partner and family if you start to feel low or anxious – share the symptoms of postnatal depression with them too, so that they know what to look out for.

3 Don't be afraid to seek help if you do have a mental health wobble – your GP is the best first port of call.

Chapter 15

Will you ever sleep again?

In the early days of twin motherhood it may well feel like you'll never get a decent night's sleep ever again. Don't panic. You will. But there's no getting away from the reality that it's going to be tough for a little while.

When it comes to sleep, I often think back to what life was like before I had kids. I'd work hard all week, often staying late in the office every night, putting in lots of hours. Sometimes on a Thursday night we'd go to the pub and after a few glasses of wine I'd get home at gone midnight and only manage a few hours of sleep before it was time to get up and get ready for work the next day. I'd spend that day feeling tired but getting work done, going to meetings, knowing that at the end of the day I could head home and collapse onto the sofa before an early night. There was always the comfort of knowing I could catch up on any missed sleep.

One of the biggest learning curves of motherhood, for me, was: There isn't going to be a chance to catch up on sleep. In those early days it really panicked me that there was no option to just have a lie in, or go to bed early, because you're always on duty – 24/7! 'It's just so relentless,' I sobbed to my husband one evening,

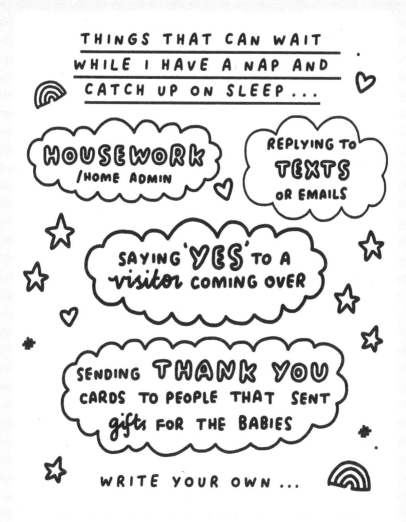

THINGS THAT CAN WAIT
WHILE I HAVE A NAP AND
CATCH UP ON SLEEP...

HOUSEWORK /HOME ADMIN

REPLYING TO TEXTS OR EMAILS

SAYING 'YES' TO A visitor COMING OVER

SENDING THANK YOU CARDS TO PEOPLE THAT SENT gifts FOR THE BABIES

WRITE YOUR OWN...

back when my eldest was only a few weeks old. So when I had my twins I was prepared for the relentless lack of sleep. And I knew that with a bit of planning we could work around it as best we could.

Because here's the reality: you need to forget any notion of sleep being a thing that you do between 11pm and 7am. When you have newborn twins, sleep is now something that you grab in snatches, whenever you can get it! Especially when you consider that newborn babies don't know the difference between day and night so, to begin with, they might be awake at night just as much as they are during the day.

I think changing the way I viewed sleep really helped me get through the fourth trimester in one piece. Unlike last time, I didn't feel anxious if I'd only managed three hours sleep in a night – in fact, I saw that as being a big win – three hours? In a block? Brilliant!

We put a plan in place to take turns doing 'shifts' throughout the night. It sounds kind of bonkers now, but it worked for us. We popped a cot in our living room and that's where the twins slept (day and night) for the first few weeks. Being in the same cot seemed to settle them better, and they slept happily through all of the usual noise that a family home creates – our eight-year-old singing and dancing, the TV being on, the radio, you name it. We were feeding the twins every three hours – and midwives advised us to carry on with this through the night, to try to get the babies putting on weight as they should be – so during the day, we'd wake them for their feed and then they'd usually fall asleep again straight away so after burping them, we'd pop them back in their cot.

5 THINGS things to try, when helping your twins to sleep well

Jo Tantum (@jotantum), baby sleep expert

1 Swaddle them Twins have been quite cosy and snug in the womb, so when they're born, they might not feel as secure. Swaddling them with a light, breathable, stretchy material can really help.

2 Use white noise and womb sounds to soothe them There can be lots of noises while your twins sleep during the day and then, at night, it can be very quiet. Playing womb sounds, while they sleep, is a great way to reassure them.

3 Have them together in a cot It can be a good idea to place them side by side – with a gap between – in a regular-sized cot (not a Moses basket). In my experience, they settle well when together and, 90 per cent of the time, if one twin is crying than the other twin will be completely oblivious.

4 Don't rush to them at every little squeak or noise It can be tempting to rush in and pick up a baby when they make little noises, but what can happen is they never get used to noise around them.

5 Wake them up for feeds during the day It's likely you'll be feeding your twins every three or four hours. I recommend you wake them up for feeds in the day – it can help with the day/night confusion. At night, unless you've been advised to wake them to feed, you can leave them to have a longer sleep. If one wakes for a feed at night, it's a good idea to wake the other so that they're on roughly the same schedule.

Our *(slightly bonkers but it worked for us)* **night-time routine**

8pm	I'd go to bed and my husband would stay with the babies in the living room.
10pm	I'd wake up and feed the babies, then my husband would go to bed and I'd sit up with the babies (and watch *Gilmore Girls*).
1am	My husband would wake up, help me feed the babies and then I'd go to bed, and he would sit up with the babies/doze on the sofa.
4am	I'd wake up and feed the babies, then my husband would go to bed and I'd sit up with the babies (and watch *Downton Abbey*).
7am	My husband would wake up, shower, help me feed the babies and then I'd go to bed, while he got our eight-year-old ready for the day.
10am	I'd get up, shower, feed the babies and would start the day properly.

I've heard of some people doing something similar where they have the babies in their nursery and they pop a mattress on the floor to allow them to sleep and tend to the babies easily. We found it worked being in the living room because we had the

TV there, the sofa to snooze on, we were close to snacks in the kitchen, and being downstairs meant the sleeping parent and our eight-year-old weren't disturbed by any crying babies!

We did this for quite a few weeks, and then moved them to our bedroom when it was clear they were going to sleep a bit longer in the night and health visitors told us we could leave them to sleep without waking them.

MY TIPS for surviving the sleep saga

 Buy an eye mask to help you sleep during the day.

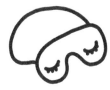

 'Sleep when the baby sleeps' is such a cliché but if you can make it work, do it. If you've got an older child who isn't at school yet, snuggle up and watch a TV show together. Rest doesn't have to be actual sleep – time sitting quietly, reading or watching TV can be restorative.

 A normal sleep cycle is 45 minutes so even if you just have a one-

hour window, it's worth grabbing it as you will wake up feeling better.

 If caffeine affects you, try cutting down or out completely (I know, sounds like terrible advice when your instinct is to drink all the coffee in the world) so that you don't find yourself lying in bed at 2pm, trying to nap, feeling a bit wired.

 Going to bed as early as you can in the evening is such a game-changer. The temptation can be to stay up and watch TV with your partner but it's a great time to get some 'bonus' sleep in.

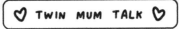

'My twins were terrible sleepers'

NICOLE, MUM TO TWO-YEAR-OLD TWINS

My girls have always been bad sleepers, since day one really. They had reflux and CMPA (allergy to cow's milk) that wasn't diagnosed until they were about four months old, which would have definitely impacted sleep problems. I breastfed on demand when they were babies and fed them to sleep but this meant every single time they woke up, I had to wake and feed.

It was almost impossible to get them to do this at the same time and my life was consumed by trying to get them to be in synch with each other. There were nights when they were both waking every 30–45 minutes but about 15–20 minutes out from each other so I was getting 15–25-minute snatches of sleep. We starting waking one twin if the other one woke and then I nearly always tandem fed, which saved time, but in the early days I found it difficult to get them both well positioned and latched on my own. It took some practice but we managed.

My husband was amazing. In the nights he used to get up with me and he would change nappies and pass babies to me and help me get comfortable then grab a few more minutes' sleep as I fed. Then I'd wake him up and he'd help with winding, any more nappy changes and trying to settle them back in bed.

Once I was fully healed from my C-section and more mobile, I started to let him sleep more as he had to get up, drive to work and work all day, whereas I could grab naps during the day when the babies slept sometimes. Surviving on not a lot of sleep was something that – before the babies – I wouldn't have believed I'd be able to do, and looking back now I don't know how I did it in that newborn stage. It's amazing what the human body can do when it comes to your children. I definitely moaned about it though! A real lifesaver was the group chat with a group of mummy friends. We'd all done pregnancy yoga together and remained friends and all our children were due within a couple of months of each other.

Between us all we really had pretty much every experience imaginable of conceiving, pregnancy, labour, feeding, sleeping etc., so we all had plenty to talk about. It was amazing at 2am to be able to reach for my phone and connect with friends who were all up and going through the same thing as me (one of the other girls also had twins so we even had that covered!). They really helped me keep some sanity in the early days – and still do now that all the babies are turning two!

The babies eventually started sleeping through the night but they are early risers and wake up for the day somewhere between 4 and 6am. The average these days is that they wake up about 5:30 and I leave them chatting until 6, but I know my first twin is the culprit who wakes her sister up! I think I have read every theory in the world about how to get babies to sleep more/longer/later in the morning but have accepted that there's not a lot you can do! The sleep deprivation has been so difficult – I said to my husband the other day that I don't think I've had a proper night's sleep since before I got pregnant so sometime in early 2017! It's hard when friends tell me how they had to wake their child up at 8:30am to leave the house and then they still have a two or three-hour nap and go to bed by seven. I just try to look on the bright side of all the extra cuddles I'm getting!

Safe sleeping for twins

Advice from The Lullaby Trust

You may like to have your twins in their own Moses baskets or cots from birth, or you may decide to co-bed them in the early weeks and months. Co-bedding means siblings share the same sleep surface during any sleep period, for example, by being in the same cot together. It can help them regulate their body temperatures and sleep cycles, and can soothe them and their twin. If you do co-bed them:

- Only place them side-by-side in a cot in the early weeks, when they can't roll over or onto each other. Make sure they are not close enough to touch and potentially obstruct each other's breathing.

- There's no need to use rolled-up towels, pillows or anything else between their heads and the use of cot dividers is not recommended. These items can become potential hazards.

- It might be good to start sleeping them at opposite ends of their cot from the beginning – this means they'll both be in the 'feet to foot' position with their own bedding firmly tucked in. You may choose instead to use sleeping bags.

- Once either of your babies have learnt to roll, it might be practical to move them to their own sleep surfaces. This is to prevent one from obstructing the breathing of the other, or causing an accident.

- It is not advisable to place your twins in the same Moses basket, even when they are very small. This is to minimise the chance of them overheating, which is known to increase the chance of SIDS. Even with small babies a Moses basket is too small for two babies to sleep safely.

IF YOU ONLY DO 3 THINGS

1 Think about whether a routine or being more baby-led might work for you.

2 Get snatches of rest or sleep whenever you can – even if it's just a short amount of time. It all adds up.

3 Download a white noise app onto your phone (there are lots of free ones).

Chapter 16

When it feels like they'll never stop crying . . .

For me, one of the most emotionally tough things about having newborn twins was the late afternoon and evening crying. Some people call it 'the witching hour' and experts say it's a real thing! Often babies are overstimulated by this time of day, there's often extra activity in the home with people arriving from work, school and nursery, and you might be feeling a bit frazzled too, which babies can pick up on.

One evening, when our twins were around four weeks old and we were in the thick of relentless evening crying, we had both of them very upset at the same time. It was around 8pm and we'd had one of them crying, on and off, for an hour or so. We tried cuddling them. 'If I hold this one in this position and rock her like this, she seems to stop crying,' I said to my husband, standing and rocking while we tried to watch an old episode of *Friends*. It was amazing. She fell asleep in my arms and I slowly sat down on the sofa with her, still rocking her. *Immediately*, as soon as I sat down, she woke up and started crying again. 'It's like she has a sixth sense, even when asleep, and knows when I've sat down!' I said to my husband, standing back up again through my incredible tiredness.

Meanwhile, he had the other twin in a bouncer chair, hoping that the gentle rocking would soothe her. Eventually, when all else failed, we got a sling each and popped a twin in. My twin settled when I took big giant steps through the kitchen, falling asleep as she nestled into my chest. And then as soon as I sat down . . . yes, you've guessed it, she woke up and cried again. That night, and plenty of other nights, it really felt like no matter what we did, one or both of the babies would be crying.

It can be so hard to stay calm when you have two screaming babies to soothe.

In fact, studies have shown that the sound of a crying baby is processed by your brain in a different way to other sounds. It activates the parts of the brain involved with emotion processing and which control our fight-or-flight response. It's almost like it's designed to make us react to it instinctively. The sound is also believed to increase oxytocin levels in us, to encourage us to give cuddles and care to our baby (but you might not feel a rush of warm love that you usually associate with oxytocin – if you're anything like me, you might just feel stressed!).

How do I know if my babies have colic?

Following what's called the Wessel Criteria, if one or both of your babies cry for more than three hours a day, for more than three days a week, for more than three weeks, they might be diagnosed by a medical professional with colic. It's common to get this confused with colic in horses, which is linked to trapped wind, but colic in babies has nothing to do with trapped wind. There's no treatment for it – it's not an actual medical diagnosis – it's just a way of describing what the baby is going through.

8 THINGS to remember
when your babies cry a lot

Sarah Ockwell-Smith (@sarahockwellsmith), parenting expert who specialises in the psychology and science of parenting, 'gentle parenting' and attachment theory

THERE WILL BE TIMES WHEN YOUR BABIES CRY AND YOU HAVE NO IDEA WHY AND THAT'S OK

You can go through the list, you know, are they hungry? Are they thirsty? Are they in pain? Are they tired? Are they uncomfortable? They will still cry, and it's important to understand this is totally normal.

GET OUTSIDE AND GO FOR A WALK

It might feel like the last thing you want to do but getting outside and getting some fresh air when your babies are crying can be so good. It can blow the cobwebs away for you, and with the babies, often the change of temperature or atmosphere or air pressure or sound, can be really good for babies and you might find they calm down.

DON'T FEEL GUILTY IF YOUR BABY CRIES A LOT

New mums can put a lot of pressure on themselves to try to understand their babies all the time. If your babies are crying lots and you don't know why, you might feel incredibly guilty and like a failure. You're not. It's something all babies do.

'THE WITCHING HOUR' IS MORE A THING FOR PARENTS THAN BABIES

We're absolutely exhausted. We've gone through the whole day, often alone as a mum, and it's common to feel like you can't take any more. And babies really do pick up on our emotions. I don't mean this to sound judgmental – because we're all doing our very best – but if you're really stressed and feel tense by the end of the day, and you perhaps start to cope less well than normal, babies somehow pick up on it and it can cause them to cry more.

JUST HOLDING YOUR BABY WHEN THEY CRY IS OFTEN THE BEST THING YOU CAN DO

What we know from science is that if you hold a baby when they're crying, they release significantly less cortisol (the stress hormone) and it impacts in different areas of their brain. So if they're crying and you're holding them, it isn't toxic and stressful for them. It doesn't have that negative impact on their brain.

TRY TO PREVENT THE CRYING RATHER THAN REACT TO IT

So if you have babies who get fractious at 4pm or 5pm, I wouldn't wait for them to get fractious and then try and soothe them. If you use a sling to soothe them, put it on at 3pm – putting a baby in a sling when he's really upset is not going to work. So if you see a pattern, try to prevent the pattern an hour before it normally happens

BE CAREFUL OF OVERSTIMULATION

There's this thing in our society where we think we have to entertain babies. So we're constantly going to different baby groups and buying all these loud brightly coloured toys. If you've got eight-week-old twins, eight weeks ago they were in the dark, with pretty much no stimulation. All of a sudden, they've got these different sights, sounds, smells, to deal with and I do think that contributes to tricky evenings.

IF END-OF-THE-DAY CRYING IS BAD, GET SOME EXTRA SUPPORT

Ask a family member if they can pop over at a certain time each day. Ideally, it'll be someone who you can just moan to, and not someone who'll say, 'Have you tried this …?' or suggest you leave the babies to cry it out. You really don't want advice. New mums get so much bloody advice from everybody! What you need is to somebody to listen and be a sounding board that you can just have a whinge at.

'I learned to accept help when my babies wouldn't stop crying'

AILIS, MUM TO ONE-YEAR-OLD TWIN GIRLS

———

My twins cried a lot when they were little. My husband went back to work full-time after three weeks and we have no family close by, so I was on my own with them most of the time. When you're home alone with them it can feel like you are the only one in that situation, but in reality, every new mum is going through the same.

At different points I tried dummies, slings, rockers, you name it! Randomly, I found that singing YMCA (the bit starting with 'Young man . . .') calmed my two when they were melting down. I have no idea what the neighbours must have thought! One particularly traumatic day when they were a couple of months old, neither would stop crying. I felt desperate and panicked. I was flustered and tearful. I didn't know what I was doing wrong. (Now I realise I was doing nothing wrong at all)! It was spring and I was in the garden. One of my neighbours came out and asked if I needed any help so I passed one of the babies over the garden fence to her! She was absolutely thrilled. She practically jumped over the fence to help! About an hour later I had a gardener (who I had never met) come over to give me a quote and I ended up handing him a baby while I settled the other! It was one of those, 'What am I doing?!' moments but also a reminder about the importance of accepting help when it's offered. That would be key piece of advice I would give to new twin mums – ask for help if you need it and definitely accept any help that's offered!

PLACES TO GO FOR ONLINE SUPPORT

❋ **Mumsnet**
mumsnet.com
The forums on Mumsnet are packed with mums chatting about everything from pregnancy, sleep deprivation and weaning to celebrities, neighbour feuds and school issues. Even old threads can be a mine of helpful information – I often google something like: 'Mumsnet swaddling tips,' to get old threads of people discussing something.

❋ **The Motherload Facebook group**
facebook.com/groups/wearethemotherload
This is one of the biggest Facebook parenting communities, and it's one of the most supportive and non-judgemental you'll find.

❋ **Your local twins group's Facebook page**
Search Facebook or Google for info on the group if you're not already aware of your local twin group. Most of them have a Facebook group for members to chat in the middle of the night and seek support when they need it.

❋ **Twins Trust's Twinline**
email asktwinline@twinstrust.org or call 0800 138 0509 Monday to Friday from 10am to 1pm and from 7pm to 10pm.
Staffed by trained volunteers who are all parents of twins, Twinline offers support and advice on any aspect of being a twin parent.

If you're feeling overwhelmed by the crying . . .

1 Get out and about
If your babies won't settle indoors, take them out for a walk. We did this, even if it was dark outside, and without fail it made me feel better. Often the babies were asleep by the time I got to the end of the road and I benefited from the endorphins from a quick walk.

2 Eat your 'main meal' at lunchtime
We found that our babies were most fractious in the evenings just as we were trying to cook – and eat – dinner. So I started eating my main meal at lunchtime (if you have some batch-cooked or donated one-pot meals it's perfect to heat up with some veg on the side). Then, in the evenings, we ate something quick and easy to prepare or snack on with one hand, like cold meat, hummus and salad. It took a bit of pressure off the evenings and gave us more time to devote to soothing the babies.

3 Take turns soothing the babies with your partner
It can feel pretty relentless so try giving each other a break. Take yourself off for a soothing lavender bath for an hour, and then give your partner a break in return.

4 Don't feel like a dummy
One popular way of soothing a crying baby is using a dummy (soother). Sucking can lower a baby's heart rate, blood pressure and stress levels. There's also evidence that suggests dummies can help prevent SIDS (Sudden Infant Death Syndrome). It's recommended that if you want to give your babies a dummy that you wait until breastfeeding is established. Of course, there's a bit of a stigma around giving your baby a dummy, but if it's something that soothes your twins (and soothes you!) then don't let the judgement of others stop you.

IF YOU ONLY DO 3 THINGS

1 Get outdoors if the crying is overwhelming - the fresh air will do you good and the change of atmosphere and noise might calm your babies.

2 Remember, it's normal for babies to cry a lot when they're young.

3 If you need to, ask for extra support - either from family or find some virtual support in online twin groups.

Chapter 17

Going it alone (*you can do it!*)

You might be in a position where your partner (if you don't have a partner, see page 227) is able to take longer than the usual, statutory two weeks' leave when you have your twins. More and more people are able to request extended parental leave, flexible working hours or working from home for part or all of the week, which can all be a huge help when getting to grips with life with twins.

But for many new twin mums, the reality will be having two weeks with your partner, working as a team, learning what your babies need and how to best deliver that. Sometimes this time can even be swallowed up caring for babies in SCBU or NICU and by the time you get the babies home, your partner is already back at work.

It can feel like it's incredibly unfair – just as you're getting into the swing of things, you suddenly have to do it *all by yourself*.

When I had my twins, I was in the incredibly fortunate – and unusual – position to have my husband around all of the time. I'm self-employed and happen to earn more than he does, so it didn't make any sense for me to take a big chunk of time off work looking

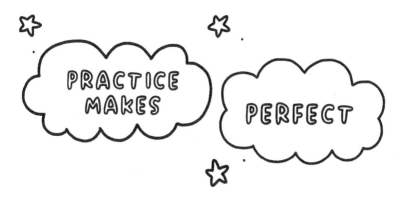

PRACTICE MAKES PERFECT

after the twins on my own and for him to carry on working full-time. Instead, he gave up work and was there to support me and our twins (and the big one!), which was amazing. Then, when the babies were a few months old, I started working again – I work from home so I could work between breastfeeds! Lots of people seem surprised that we did it this way, but it's pretty much the same as every other couple, we just swapped the usual roles of mum staying at home with babies, dad going back to work. My husband is still a stay-at-home dad to our girls and I'm now working full-time.

But that said, I know what a shock to the system it can be when your partner goes back to work from when our first daughter was a baby. In those two weeks, I grew to rely on the help he was giving me. Just having someone around to make me a sandwich, pass me the TV remote while I was breastfeeding and to keep checking in with me on whether I was drinking enough water, was invaluable. In fact, I don't think I even appreciated how much I needed that help until – POOF – one Monday at 7.30am, it walked out of the door wearing a shirt and tie.

For two weeks we'd been a team, making joint decisions on when to feed the baby, how best to burp the baby, working out why she was crying, working out why I was crying, taking turns to do the night shift while the other one slept.

But on that morning, when it was time for him to go back to work, the realisation hit me. The front door banged shut, signalling that I was suddenly, truly, alone with my 14-day-old baby. I remember looking at the clock on the oven: 7.35am. Then I looked at my baby, dozing in my arms, and sheer panic washed over me. How the flip was I going to do this on my own? How was I going to take a shower? How would I have time to go to the loo? What if I left the house on my own, forgetting I even had a baby?

Of course, it was fine. I got through that day, and the next, and the next, in one piece. But that mental transition from being able to rely on someone else to help you navigate each tiny task to doing it alone felt huge. I won't lie to you and say I found it easy. I didn't. It was hard being at home on my own with a baby that was too small to chat back to me. I felt lonely and even though he was having to go to work every day feeling knackered from the broken sleep, I envied my husband being able to sit on the train for half an hour as he commuted to work. I envied him for being able to chat to his colleagues across the desk (at that time he worked in an office). And I really bloody envied him being able to drink cups of hot coffee and wander to Leon to buy meatballs at lunchtime. My husband, thankfully, did everything he could to make it easier for me: texting me throughout the day to ask how we were, offering support when I was having a bad day, leaving the office bang on 5pm each day and not even thinking about asking if he could go to the pub with his workmates.

I think it would have really helped to have someone sit me down and say: It won't feel this hard forever. It feels hard right now, because you're suddenly doing it all by yourself. But you'll soon be changing nappies one-handed, packing a change bag with your eyes closed and the thought of having to fold up the buggy on your own won't bring you out in a cold sweat. Practice makes perfect, right? And even better: no one's expecting perfection from you!

A NOTE TO SEND YOUR FAMILY + FRIENDS!

Dear ....,

WHEN .... GOES BACK TO WORK, I'M GOING TO NEED SOME MORE HELP WITH THE TWINS. I'D LOVE IT IF YOU WOULD BE UP FOR COMING OVER TO LEND A HAND. THE KINDS OF THINGS I COULD REALLY DO WITH SOME HELP WITH ARE:

....

....

....

(SUGGESTIONS) MAKING ME CUPS OF TEA, MAKING ME LUNCH, HELPING ME WITH FEEDING THE BABIES, RUNNING AROUND WITH THE VACUUM CLEANER.

Love ....

x ♡ x

MY TOP TIPS FOR WHEN YOUR PARTNER GOES BACK TO WORK

* Talk about your feelings before your partner goes back to work. It's OK to admit that you're feeling anxious about it.

* Make a plan for that first week – even if it just involves which box sets you'll watch and who will come to visit you.

* Try to get out and about a little – a walk to your local park for some fresh air is ideal.

* Keep in touch with your partner throughout the day.

* Remember, it's not easy for your partner either.

* Don't try to do it all – the housework and cooking can still be divided between you and your partner.

* Practise feeding the babies on your own before you have to, so that it's not something you're worried about doing.

* Have a nappy changing 'station' in your living room so that you can easily change one nappy without leaving the other baby.

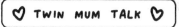

'Looking after twins and a toddler was hard – but I did it!'

**BROOKE, MUM TO TWO-YEAR-OLD TWINS
AND FOUR-YEAR-OLD SINGLETON**

My twin boys were born at 36 weeks, and I had a toddler too. My partner took two weeks off – actually, he took one week off, then went back for a few days because we knew I'd have lots of family flocking to visit me, and then he took another week off. So I had three weeks of having that support, which was great. But from the day my partner went back to work, it was pretty much just me and the boys. My mum would come over once a week to help for the day – I really relied on her to clean – but for 90 per cent of the time, it was just me and the boys.

It was exhausting. It really was. Keeping busy helped, so we carried on taking my eldest to toddler group. I think I always thought: it could get harder, but they're babies right now and we can do this. I had one in the carrier, one in the buggy and it worked! I think I was a lot more relaxed, having done it before, so I knew what I'd need for a trip out with them – do we need four outfits? No! It was easier to streamline things.

I was just so much more willing to accept help with the twins too. Also, I think maybe I was a bit defiant, in a way. I wanted to prove that I could handle having three little children! When I was pregnant, so many people were shocked it was twins and said, 'Oh, what are you going to do?' and, 'Oh, it's going to be so hard' and it was, but it wasn't! I think you just have to get on with it.

Survive going it alone with a smile!

Beccy Hands (@beccyhands), doula and postnatal massage expert

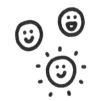

CREATE A ROTA WITH FAMILY MEMBERS

When your partner goes back to work is when you need some extra support. So it can be a good idea to stave people off in the first two weeks while your partner is at home by saying, 'I would really love to have your help when they're back at work. Can I book you for a whole day or an afternoon or a morning?' You can schedule people in for two or three weeks and even just being able to visually see that support in your diary can make things feel easier.

BOOK IN FRIENDS TO HELP, TOO

Rather than inviting people to come and meet the babies, if you slightly reframe the way you're talking, like, 'I know I'm going to need a bit scooping up, so if you wouldn't mind coming and spending the afternoon with me?' then people are (usually!) suddenly all, 'Of course!' People love to support and, you know, it's quite an honour to be asked. So send a clear message that you're booking them in to help.

IF YOU DON'T HAVE FAMILY AND FRIENDS NEARBY, HIRE A POSTNATAL DOULA

(See page 183 for more on doulas.)

DON'T TRY TO GET THE HOUSEWORK DONE OR ACHIEVE MUCH AT ALL WHILE YOU'RE AT HOME WITH TWINS

When your partner gets home, you can either hand them a list of stuff to do, or – because you've been with the babies all day – you might want to hand them over and then go and do stuff in the kitchen or around the home because it gives you a break from the babies!

PLAN YOUR FOOD FOR THE NEXT DAY

Some days are all right and some days are just an absolute write off and you're not going to get anything done, so if you can, make some breakfast muffins, make yourself a sandwich – you can even make up a packed lunch in a box with a sandwich, some chopped-up veg or a big pot of hummus and a huge tub of crudites that you can graze on throughout the day. Imagine you're going out the next day and you're making three meals to take with you.

ORGANISE ANYTHING YOU'RE GOING TO NEED FOR THE NEXT DAY

Lay out a change of clothes for each of the babies, lay the nappy-changing station out ready, re-pack your change bag with nappies and anything you might need so that the next morning that's all ready to go.

BEFORE YOUR PARTNER LEAVES FOR WORK, GET THEM TO MAKE YOU A SMOOTHIE

Because then even if you do live on toast for the rest of the day, you've got loads of nutrients already from that smoothie. You can prepare them ahead of time – get freezer bags and chop all your ingredients up, put them in the bag and freeze them. Then it's just a case of tipping it in a blender with whatever milk or yogurt you're using. So quick and easy!

If you're going it alone 24/7

For those mums who are doing this by themselves, through choice or circumstance, the advice is simple: get as much support as you can. Appoint one or two family members or friends as your 'key support' – make sure it's people who you know you can really count on to be there for you. You'll soon get into the swing of things, and will be able to do everything by yourself, but at the start extra support will be invaluable.

Beccy's favourite smoothies for new mums

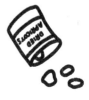

If you're breastfeeding	If you need an iron boost	If you need one with diuretic powers (*great for flushing out excess fluids*)
1 banana 120g oats 2 tablespoons peanut butter 1 tablespoon brewer's yeast 2 tablespoons cacao powder 1 teaspoon vanilla extract 1 tablespoon milled flaxseed 1 tablespoon maple syrup 250ml milk or coconut milk	1 handful spinach ½ avocado 1 handful kale Small handful blueberries Small bunch mint leaves 1 tablespoon flaxseed 1 tablespoon chia seeds 250ml water 3 dried apricots 3 dates (stones removed)	250ml apple juice 225g pineapple chunks 1 handful watercress 1 celery stick 1 handful grapes 1 handful blueberries

FOR MORE SMOOTHIE RECIPES, SEE *THE LITTLE BOOK OF SELF-CARE FOR NEW MUMS* BY BECCY HANDS AND ALEXIS STICKLAND

IF YOU ONLY DO 3 THINGS

1 Get family members and friends involved – book them in to help you.

2 Don't even attempt to do housework or get life admin done to start with.

3 Organise what you'll need for the following day – meals, outfits, clean nappies, the lot!

Chapter 18

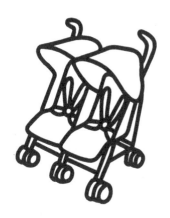

Getting out and about

The first time that I took my twins out on my own I was filled with worry.

* *What if they both need changing at the same time?*

* *What if they need feeding while we're out? Tandem breastfeeding or bottle-feeding two babies at the same time is tricky, right?!*

* *What if they both start crying while we're out?*

* *What if we need to get on a bus and I can't fit my double buggy on?*

* *If we're going out in the car, is it OK to leave one baby-in-car-seat in the house while I take the first baby-in-car-seat out to the car?*

* *What if I forget something like the rain covers or spare nappies?*

I was on my own with them, and wanted to get out of the house to buy a few supermarket essentials. 'Right, girls,' I said to them, enthusiastically. 'We're going to drive to the big supermarket.'

They said nothing in response . . . because they were only a couple of months old. But they kicked their legs happily on their playmat, which I took to be a sign of being up for this pivotal trip out.

I packed their change bag with everything I might need and strapped them into their car seats. The fact that I managed to put their car seats into the car correctly felt like a huge achievement. I parked the car at the supermarket – securing a rare parent-and-child parking space – and was able to unfold the double buggy (something I hadn't done previously, without being reminded which bit to press, which part to pull and which section to swing up), I managed to put the car seat extensions on the buggy (this might have taken around ten minutes while I faffed over which one was the left and which one was the right) and finally popped the car seats onto the buggy, ready to wheel into the supermarket. Success!

They both seemed quite happy, so once I'd got my groceries I even braved having a little wander around the clothing section. It felt exhilarating! I was out! On my own! With my twin babies!

As you might expect, one of them needed a nappy change, and instead of panicking, I calmly wheeled them into the baby change room, changed the nappy and headed out. Driving home, I felt so proud of myself. It may sound like such a small, silly thing to be proud of, but I'd managed it! I'd gone out with the babies by myself and I'd coped. There's no reason why you can't get out and about with your twins, if you want to.

Your <u>step-by-step</u> plan to getting out with your twins

Day 1	Start small by going for a walk around the block.
Day 2	Go one step further and pop to your local shop – negotiating a small shop with a double pram (or single pram and sling) isn't always easy, but you can do it!
Day 3	Head further afield. Is there a cafe you can head to to meet a friend for a cuppa?
One day soon...	At some point, driving somewhere or getting on public transport is an achievement to tick off, but these are all things you can do gradually. It's not a race.

Going out with your twins is such a good thing to do – it allows you to get fresh air, get some endorphins released in your body and will help you feel like you're getting into a bit of a normal routine. It's such a good thing to do for your mental health. It's also good to get confident being out with them in case you need to take them to the GP or have any kind of an emergency that means you have to take them out.

Lots of new mums find going to a baby class or playgroup can be a good way to get out and meet other mums. There are lots of twin groups around the UK too, and it's a brilliant way to find other twin mums to chat to and share knowledge with!

Going to a baby class or group on your own can feel daunting though – one twin mum I know arranged to go with another mum friend each week so that she knew she had support if she needed it. Another twin mum told me that she always gets to her class early, and positions herself next to the teacher so that she can help her if she needs it. When you go out with twins, you realise how many people are happy to help you.

THINGS YOU MIGHT WANT TO PACK WHEN YOU HEAD OUT ON YOUR OWN

(stick the list on the fridge to help you remember!)

☐ Wipes

☐ Change of clothes

☐ Nappy bags

☐ Muslins

☐ Spare dummies/comforters

☐ Sterilised bottles with water and formula if bottle-feeding

☐ Spare nappies

5 THINGS that can help you get out the door

Alexis Stickland (@candidmidwife), midwife and postnatal author

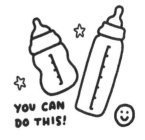

YOU CAN DO THIS!

1 **Prepare!** If you know you have to get out of the door for an appointment or you're meeting a friend the following day, get your change bag packed the night before. Get bottles sterilised and prepped, get spare baby clothes packed. If you have a partner present, get them to help.

2 **Expect that things will take longer.** Babies will poo and need feeding, they'll start crying just as you're trying to leave. Set your phone alarm for 30 minutes before you have to leave to give you lots of time to get ready and so you're not too overwhelmed by trying to get out the door on time.

3 **Don't fall into the trap of people-pleasing.** If this outing is not something you want or need to do, don't put unnecessary pressure on yourself. Stay at home and eat biscuits while watching Netflix instead! Cut yourself a break – it really is OK if you have to cancel last minute because you're on your knees with tiredness, your babies are fractious or it just all feels like too much. Remember the saying: 'When I say no to you, I say yes to me!'

4 **Understand that other people might change plans and it is not the end of the world.** Keep some perspective! Appointments can be rescheduled and meet-ups can be planned for another day.

5 **Lower your expectations significantly because then the only way is up!** Get your twins fed, changed and loved – anything extra is a bonus. You are a human being and you are doing the best you can in that moment.

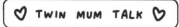

'*I had zero confidence taking my boys out alone, until a friend challenged me to do it*'

EMMA, MUM TO NON-IDENTICAL 18-MONTH-OLD TWINS

When my boys were a few months old, I was still really struggling with my confidence and taking them out on my own. It was just so overwhelming.

I'd got chatting to some other twin mums on Instagram – just by searching the #twinmum hashtag. One of them set me a challenge. She said to me, 'Emma, you need to go outside and feed the boys on your own. Get up. Throw some jogging bottoms on. I want you to go to your closest coffee shop and you need to feed the boys on your own in public'. So I did. I got the boys in the buggy and I went five minutes down the road to a coffee shop. I was so anxious – I cried on the way there, I had butterflies and I remember being really jittery as I ordered my cup of tea. But honestly, it's the best thing I did. There were lots of people there happy to help. So there was me thinking I was going to be on my own, in this crowded room, and I was going to be made to feel like a crap mum. But actually it got me out and talking to people, and I had loads of helping hands.

From that day, I made it my routine. I'd get up, get ready and go to the coffee shop with the boys, where I'd feed them and have a cup of tea. Once I'd overcome my fear, I knew I could do it. I had such a sense of pride because I got through it. My advice would be to have a practice run when your partner is at home. Also, practise feeding your twins on your own so that you can do it confidently.

Surviving immunisations day with twins

One of the toughest hurdles in these early twin motherhood days is the immunisations. They usually happen at eight weeks, 12 weeks and 16 weeks, so often it's once your partner is back at work.

I find immunisations day really tough, but I always forget how emotionally hard it is! As we walked into the small nurses' room at our local GP surgery, I found myself making ultra-chatty and bright chit-chat with the nurse, as if that would set the tone for the whole appointment. (My brain: If we're super nice to the nurse, maybe the injections won't hurt?)

But while I stripped off a baby, I could feel my heart rate increasing and as I gripped her leg tightly ('Hold it really tight, Mum,' the nurse was instructing me), tears welled up in my eyes. As the injections happen, it's the baby's screams that get you – the confused screams!

And the worst thing about that day? We then had to immediately do it all over again with the second twin! Strip, grip, cry, cuddle. There aren't many times in life when you purposefully do something that will hurt and upset your small child, are there? It feels so awful. But here are some things you can do to make the day a little less awful . . .

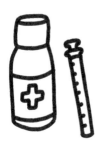

* **Make sure you take someone with you** – either get your partner to take a day off work or ask a family member or friend. It's useful to have someone there to hold one baby while you're stripping, holding for injections and dressing the other. It's also good to have a second person there to listen to the things the nurse is telling you.

* **Check with your surgery whether they recommend you give Calpol to the babies before the appointment or not** – for some vaccinations, they do. (Calpol can be given to babies aged over 2–3 months for post-vaccination fever, as long as they weigh over 4kg and were not premature.)

* **If you can, book the appointment on a day when you have nothing else on.** The babies might be feeling a bit rubbish afterwards but so might you! The best thing you can do afterwards is go home for a big cup of tea and cuddles.

* **When you put the appointment in your diary**, write in '*THIS MIGHT BE AN EMOTIONALLY TOUGH DAY!*' as a reminder to be extra kind to yourself.

* **Consider getting the following 'Vaccination day kit' in:**
    * **Calpol** (for the babies)
    * **Tissues** (for you and the babies!)
    * **Cake** (for you, after the appointment)
    * **Wine** (for you, that evening)

* **Dress your little ones in a really easy outfit** – top and leggings/joggers or a onesie – so that getting them dressed again afterwards is as stress-free as possible.

* **Be ready to just go with the flow for the next 24 hours.** Your babies might not have any side effects from the immunisations but they could get a temperature.

THE THINGS YOU'LL HEAR FROM PEOPLE WHILE YOU'RE OUT WITH YOUR TWINS...

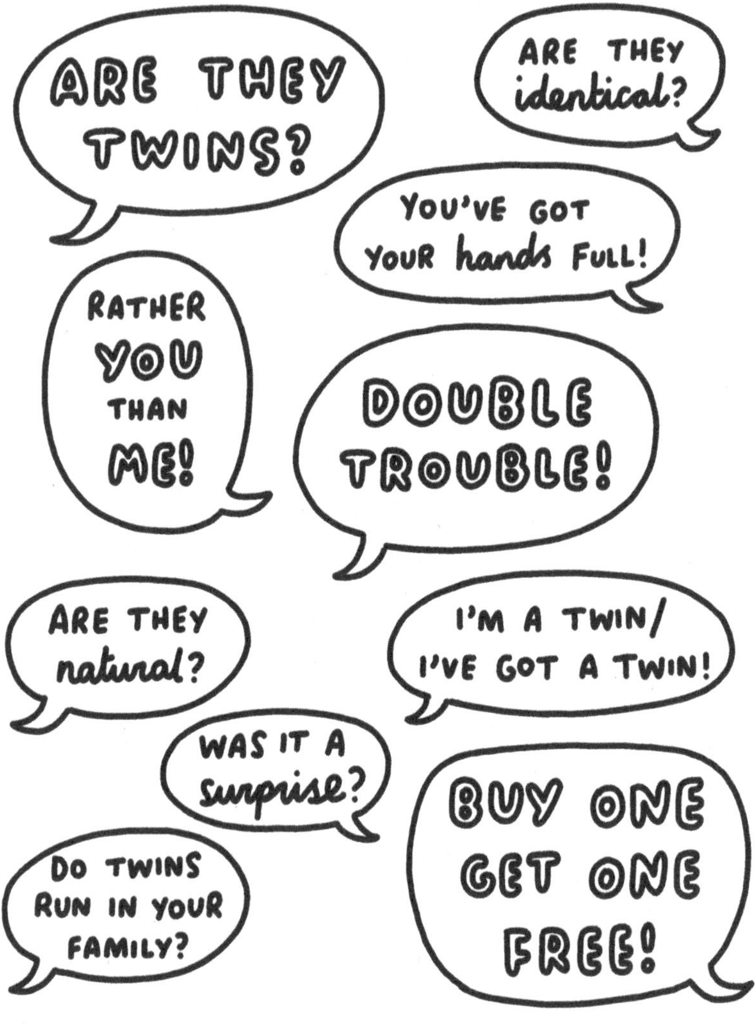

IF YOU ONLY DO 3 THINGS

1 Take things at your own pace. You don't have to be booking yourself into baby classes and meeting friends for lunch in week one of being by yourself.

2 Get fresh air every day if you can. Even if it's just walking around the block with the pram.

3 Stick a checklist of things to pack on your fridge.

Chapter 19

Your new twin mum identity

When you become a mum for the first time, something shifts inside you and it never changes back. You start to see the world in a totally different way. Your whole identity changes and it was something that I really struggled with when I first became a mum. Part of this is hormonal – described as 'matrescence' in the 1970s by American anthropologist Dana Raphael (who also coined the term, 'doula'). Similar in ways to adolescence, matrescence is when hormonal and physical shifts affect how you view the world and force you to analyse how you fit into the world.

When I first became a mum, there was never a question that it was my biggest achievement – far bigger than any professional accomplishment. But everyone suddenly viewed me differently (and I was different!) but I didn't like it. I fought the urge to post every little update about my baby on Facebook ('*I don't want to become a baby bore.*'), I still wore trendy clothes (the confused looks I got from other mums when I turned up to baby sensory class wearing an animal hat . . . hey, Katy Perry and Rihanna were wearing them, the other mums just didn't realise how cutting-edge I was), and I still wanted to make it to my friends' birthday drinks in the pub, so would take a breast pump and sit in the loos expressing milk before joining them for a glass of Sauvignon Blanc. I guess I wanted to be seen as one of those mums who just

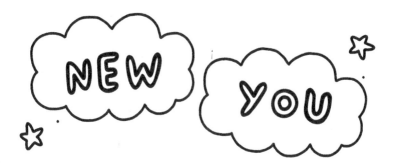

NEW YOU

happened to have a baby. 'Oh what, me? Yeah, I have a baby. But I'm totally the same person as I was before.'

Except I wasn't. Yet there I was, battling against 'mum' becoming a big part of my identity, with all the strength I had. Which isn't surprising when you think about the negative connotations that motherhood often has in society.

Lauren Laverne sums this up well, writing for the now-defunct online magazine *The Pool*: 'In our cultural conversation, "mum" is a diminished status, often preceded by the qualifier "just a",' she writes. 'Pregnancy, birth and (most of all) post-pregnancy is horrifying. Mothers are encouraged to cling onto or reclaim their pre-children lives – to get their bodies "back" after having a baby. The best compliment you can give a pregnant woman is to tell her she looks tiny. The nicest thing you can say to a new mother is that she doesn't look like she's had a baby at all. If "being a woman is the ultimate insult," it follows that being a mother isn't too far behind.'

But once I'd accepted that motherhood had changed me forever – and in ways I could never have predicted (I couldn't watch anything too violent or dystopian on TV, for example, almost like I was desperate to see the world as a good, decent place for my child to grow up in) – I started to enjoy it more. I allowed myself to post online about my baby; I developed a confidence around being a mum and being proud of it.

But if first-time motherhood gives you a whole new identity, it's nothing compared with becoming a twin mum. Becoming a twin mum allows you access into an exclusive club. I'll be walking down the street with my double pram, spot a mum with a double buggy and we'll both nod and smile. It's like we're acknowledging the hard work (and amazing times) that the other has gone through.

I've lost count of the number of shop assistants or waitresses who have told me they have twins or that they *are* a twin! Honestly, I think I've met every twin there is in my local area.

Not only that, *other people* who don't have twins will treat you like you're something special, as they stand behind you in the supermarket queue. 'Oh, are they twins?!' is how the clearly delighted person usually starts the conversation. In contrast with how I felt when I was a new mum of one, I *lapped* this up. In fact, I actively encouraged it. I practically walked up and down the bakery aisle shouting: 'I've got twins! Look!'

There's almost a badge of honour that goes with the job – yes, I've got twins, and no, I don't know *how* I manage, but I do and *look,* I'm still smiling!

THINGS I *loved* ABOUT MY pre-twin LIFE...

♡♡

I FEEL **DIFFERENT** NOW BECAUSE...

✩
✩✩

THINGS I'D *like to* **STILL BE** EVEN THOUGH I'M A *twin mum*...	THINGS I'D *like to* **STILL DO** EVEN THOUGH I'M A *twin mum*...

(THE *good news* IS, YOU CAN BE + DO *whatever* YOU LIKE.)

'Becoming a twin mum totally changed my identity''

FANNY, MUM TO TWO-YEAR-OLD TWINS

———————

When you have twins, it becomes the most interesting thing about you! So whoever you're talking to, and however it comes up that you've got twins, that's all they want to talk about. I've got an older son as well and if I'm out with all three of them, he never gets a hello or anything. Everyone's just all about the babies! I mean, they're a really important part of the family, but they're not the whole thing. And in terms of my identity, I've found myself almost thinking that I have to be this super mum because I'm a twin mum. People ask, 'How do you do it?' And say, 'Oh, I couldn't do it! I'm glad it's you not me!' And then suddenly I feel like I have to be this organised, in control, prepared-for-anything mum.

I'd say, make your identity as a twin mum what you want it to be. If you want to have it as a badge of honour, and your magic power is that you were able to create two babies, then do it! If that helps lift you up when things are rough, then do that. But it's not all you are. You had a whole life before you had twin babies – and you might have had one or more children before them – and you were interesting then too. So maybe think about the things that were important to you before you had them. And you might find that they're not important anymore, but if they are, try to make time for them.

How becoming a twin mum changes your identity

Heather Dilks-Hopper, clinical psychologist and twin mum

Even if you've had a baby before, when you have twins, your identity changes

You're learning how to do this thing that you didn't know how to do before. There's something about how the babies are so dependent on you and there's no break from it. It's not like getting a new job where you can go home and say, 'Whew, that was a tough day!' You know, they're always there! So I do think your identity changes because you have to put so much of yourself to one side. And that probably happens even more when you have twins because you have to put even more of yourself to one side, you're left with so little space for yourself.

If your babies are born premature, your identity will shift with that too

My twins were born nine weeks prematurely and spent six weeks in special care. So my first six weeks as a mum were spent sitting next to a plastic box. For a lot of twin parents, to start with, their identity shifts to being the parent of a premature baby. When you're on the postnatal ward and everybody's carrying a baby around and you don't have one to carry around, your identity is 'the mum who doesn't have her babies with her.' People don't know your story, and they might feel awkward about talking to you. And then you might have to go home without your babies, if they're in SCBU and neighbours are probably spotting you and they can see you don't have your babies. That's a really weird experience.

It might take months to feel like yourself again

It certainly took me a long time before I could come up for a breath after having my twins. I reckon it was a good six months before I thought, 'Oh, I think I might feel like myself again.' Give yourself time to adjust to being a twin mum.

Try to ignore negative twin comments!

When you take your twins out, everybody comments on them. It did make me feel special, but it's surprising how many of the comments can be negative – I don't think people mean them to be negative – but I got a lot of: 'Gosh, you've got your hands full,' or, 'Double trouble!' One day, though, I walked past a building site with my twins and a builder said, 'How lucky are you? They look wonderful. You're doing a great job!' It was so lovely to hear some positivity and praise.

It's so important to connect with other twin mums

Whether it's through an antenatal class, online or through a twins club. Just having someone to go to a cafe with, and if your twins are noisy or screaming, at least there's somebody else there who understands. I think having a connection, even with just one other person who has twins, makes a difference.

Online groups can be a place that you can perhaps admit those difficult feelings

And you can see that other people might be having a hard time with the same things as you.

I think having twins is something that's quite glorified. And it is lovely but you get so many people saying, 'Oh twins! You're so lucky!' and if you're not feeling that lucky in that moment, or you're so sleep-deprived it's hard to feel lucky, it's nice to see that other people find it hard too.

IF YOU ONLY DO 3 THINGS

1 Give yourself the space to feel different to how you felt before you had your twins. It's a huge life change and it's OK to feel like your identity has shifted.

2 Connect with other twin mums – they know how you are feeling and what you're experiencing.

3 Enjoy any praise you get for being a twin mum. You deserve it!

Chapter 20

It's a family affair
(How this affects the people around you)

There is no one more affected by having twins than you – you grew them! You carried them for nine months! (OK, possibly fewer.) You gave birth to them! You have recovered – in body and mind – from the whole experience!

But that doesn't mean that it doesn't affect the people around you too. This is usually going to be your partner and (if you have any) existing children, most of all. It's important to be mindful that this *huge and intense* life moment can be a big change for them.

For any older siblings, it's a good idea to prepare them for the arrival of twins. It can be so hard on kids when there are suddenly two babies taking up everyone's attention and time. We chatted to our daughter all throughout my pregnancy about the arrival of her little sisters.

'Do you think your sisters will like pasta as much as you do?' I would ask over dinner, as she munched her spaghetti. If one of them kicked, I'd call her over to have a feel of my tummy, which she loved. We'd chat about how she could play with them. 'I'm going to play catch with them,' she'd say excitedly, before we'd explain that for a long time the babies would be zero fun to play with. 'They'll probably just lie there, kicking their legs and squawking for the first year,' I'd say to her. We talked about how much time Mummy and Daddy would have to spend looking after them, and how we might not be going on holiday the following year – in a way, we painted the picture to be more negative than it was, in a bid to manage her expectations a bit. She was so excited about them being born we didn't want her to feel like it was all a huge anticlimax.

Once they were here, we made an effort to involve our eldest in things. She'd be asked to fetch nappies for us and got loads of praise for being super helpful. Being that bit older, she even got to hold them from time to time, which was useful for us to have another pair of hands. As much as we let her help, we were careful to be guided by her – there were a few times I'd ask for help and she'd say she'd rather carry on watching TV, and that was fine. And she watched a *lot* of TV in those early days – I have zero guilt about the amount of screen time she had. The babies arrived just before her half-term holidays, which would usually be filled with days out and fun activities, but this time, there was a lot of telly and we arranged some play dates at her friends' homes to stop her from going completely stir crazy!

A few weeks after the twins had been born, we'd just moved to four-hourly feeds (having that extra hour between feeds felt like such a treat) and I decided to take my eldest out for lunch – just me and her – to spend some time together. So, straight after the late-morning feed ('I'm done feeding and burping them! Get your shoes on! Go go go!'), we headed to a local cafe. It felt surreal to be walking along the street with just an eight-year-old by my side and no pram to push! But it was brilliant – we sat eating lunch and chatting about school, about her friends, about anything she wanted.

After that, my husband and I made an effort to take her out and spend time with her each weekend – going to the park, seeing a kids' film at the cinema or popping out to spend her pocket money – and we could tell she loved having that one-on-one time with us. We were particularly aware that she'd gone from being an only child to being one of three, and wanted her to know that she is just as important as they are – even if it felt like we were spending pretty much *all of our time* looking after (and talking about) her little sisters.

A great time to make her aware of this was when we were all out together as a family. 'Oh twins! How wonderful! How old are they? Are the identical? Are they hard work?' would be the familiar conversation starter as we queued in the shop. 'It is hard work,' I'd reply, 'but thankfully they've got a *really helpful and brilliant* older sister!' Bringing her into the conversation, while praising her at the same time, helped reaffirm what an important part of the family she still was.

Carving out some time with your older children each day can work well too. I'd sit for ten minutes with my eldest while she did her homework, or I'd ask her to read some of her latest Harry Potter book to me while we snuggled under a blanket.

With all of the disruption that two new baby siblings bring, it's a great idea to stick to any routine that your older children have – so any clubs or playgroups they go to, if you can still get to them, do. (Within reason, of course, and you're absolutely allowed to press pause on any activities that you're struggling to get to!) You can always get a family member or friend to take them if you can – and the bonus of this is, it'll give you some quiet time with the babies.

HOW TO smoothly transition the family when twins arrive

Dr Katie Wood, clinical psychologist specialising in twins

OLDER SIBLINGS MIGHT FEEL DISPLACED

In my practice, I see a lot of twins and also work with the broader family to help support them. It's common for the older sibling to experience a feeling of being displaced because the focus very quickly becomes these two individuals who are a novelty. I am the sister of twins and I spent a lot of time trying to infiltrate their special bond!

EMOTIONALLY PREPARE THEM AS MUCH AS YOU CAN

Depending on their age the format that takes might look different. If you don't, some older siblings will act out. They might regress or internalise it and keep it inside. But if you prepare them, they can get used to what it means to have two new babies come along. Talk to them as much as you can in the prenatal period.

BE AVAILABLE TO THE OLDER CHILD

The impact of twins arriving, environmentally, is that the parents have much less time. They're much less available. And that's true of any older sibling, but it's accentuated in the case of twins because the parents' time is all focused on meeting the needs of these two babies. Carve out some time to spend with them.

MAKE FRIENDS WITH OTHER TWIN FAMILIES

Twin clubs can be a great place to go for extra support, and if the older sibling meets other older siblings of twins, they have that extra support too.

5 ACTIVITIES to do with an older sibling

1 **Sit with them in a quiet corner** – in a different room to the babies – and read with them.

2 **Go out for a walk with them** Make it more fun by turning it into a scavenger hunt and looking for twigs, stones, leaves and other treasure.

3 **Draw each other** – ask your older child to sit opposite you and draw you, while you draw them.

4 **Do a jigsaw puzzle together** – if you have somewhere out-of-the-way to keep the jigsaw, start a really big one and do a little bit of it each day.

5 **Start a journal together** – they can write or draw, stick stuff in, whatever they like, but encourage them to express how they feel in their journal and chat to you about it.

Your relationship with your partner

But it's not just siblings that need a bit of extra care and attention when you have twins – your relationship with your partner does too. Now, this isn't me saying you should jump back in the sack with your partner. At all. Sex is likely the last thing you want to think about right now. But it can be really easy to fall into a pattern of just seeing your partner as, and treating them like, a bit of a workmate. It's not surprising – you've both got this huge job to nail together. You're both on a learning curve, working out how this twin parent thing works, you're sleep-deprived, so any thoughts of romance or showing your love or appreciation can go firmly out of the window.

You're also far more likely to have arguments – whether it's silly squabbles over which size of nappy to buy or big dramatic fallouts – lack of sleep and the hormones still racing around your body can be to blame. So try to make (even a little bit of) time for each other – just like you might make time for older siblings.

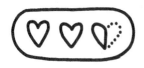

<u>HOW TO</u> make time for your relationship when you've just had twins

Susannah Baker (@one_retreat), couples therapist and founder of One Retreat

It's OK to want to be cared for and looked after (rather than desired and wanted)

This is entirely normal and OK – especially in those first few months after birth. Whatever you feel, it is vital that you can accept where your mind and body are at, and know to treat yourself with tenderness and care. This time will pass and you will feel different again.

Give each other time and space

I'm talking here to the partner who hasn't just given birth – take the babies so your partner can have a long bath, or get on with dinner unasked. Take the babies out for a walk to let her have a cup of tea and rest. These things can help the mum to feel just as loved (if not more so) as saying it out loud.

Be aware of how you each like to give and receive love

On the couples retreats I run, we talk about the 'five languages of love'. There's an online quiz at **5lovelanguages. com** that you can take at any point in your relationship (perhaps it's not one for doing when you've just had twins though!). The five languages are – 'words of affirmation,' 'acts of service,' 'quality time,' 'physical touch' and 'receiving gifts'. It's amazing how different we can be with how we like to give and receive love – my husband can clean the kitchen all day long, but it's only when he touches me that I feel loved. Knowledge of each other's top two love languages in this new post-birth period, and onwards, could really make a difference to both of you in expressing love in a language you both understand and, more importantly, *feel*. If you or your partner's top love language is 'physical touch', don't assume because you are both exhausted that intimacy cannot feature. This is the time for tenderness; for soft, affirming words, and light non-sexual touch to your partner's face, arms, hands, hair and leg.

If 'words of affirmation' are an important thing then soft, affirming words and encouragement on how amazing your partner is, spoken through the day and last thing at night, could really make a difference to their sense of wellbeing. Write a card, send surprise texts. Remind them they are loved.

'Quality time' with each other might look slightly different in this context, but if you can steal quality moments with each other, like watching a box set while doing feeds, that could also mean a lot.

'Acts of service' and 'gifts' are easy ones! Cups of tea, cooking dinner unasked, tidying up, having fresh flowers delivered, making homemade bakes, anticipating their needs, bathing the babies, changing nappies, buying your partner's favourite treat foods... the list can go on. This one is an easy win!

Pay attention to what your partner is telling you, either verbally or non-verbally

Psychologist John Gottman has some really interesting research findings on something he calls 'bids for emotional connection'. He describes these bids as attempts from one partner to another for attention, affirmation or affection. They can be either verbal or non-verbal cues and often have a secondary deeper meaning that lies beneath them.

A few examples of verbal cues:

♡ I love you

♡ Do you think this top looks OK on me?

♡ I liked it when you brought me that coffee today

Non-verbal cues could be:

♡ Slumping onto the sofa as both babies are crying uncontrollably and catching the eye of your partner with an expression of 'remember our old life?'

♡ Touching your partner's back while they stand at the hob and stir the evening meal.

♡ Reaching out to hold your partner's hand while walking along.

♡ When a baby wakes in the night, squeezing the arm of your partner as you swing your legs out of the bed, signalling that: 'I've got this.'

THINGS I'D LOVE
from MY PARTNER...

....

....

....

....

THINGS I CAN DO
for MY PARTNER...

....

....

....

....

The subtext of verbal and non-verbal cues is often something along the lines of: *'Are you with me?'*, *'Do I matter to you?'*, *'Notice me'* or *'I want to be with you'.* When our partner makes an emotional bid towards us there are three main ways in which we can respond:

- *We can turn towards them by positively responding*

- *We can turn away from them by largely ignoring them*

- *We can turn against them by actively rejecting or pushing back*

The analogy that Gottman uses is that bids can be considered within the context of an emotional bank account – you can either make deposits or withdrawals into that account. The magic ratio for this, he says, is 5 to 1. We need to have five times as much positive feeling and behaviour with our partners as negative. Small, intentional moments, like getting up to soothe a baby in the middle of the night, hold more weight than isolated, extravagant gestures when it comes to the emotional health of our relationships.

 Remember to turn towards one another and be kind
At this time when emotions are raw, life is precious and tender and you are feeling your way together as new parents, remember what brought you together in the first place and be kind to each other.

IF YOU ONLY DO 3 THINGS

1 Emotionally prepare any older siblings before the twins arrive.

2 Carve out time to spend with older siblings.

3 Pay attention to what your partner is telling you (verbally and non-verbally).

Chapter 21

The fun ahead . . .

When my twins were newly born, lots of twin mums told me that it gets easier. It was so reassuring to hear that, despite everything feeling very hard at that point, things would ease off. 'When they're a bit older, they'll be able to play with each other and you'll be able to sit back with a hot cup of tea!' one mum friend told me. 'They'll always have a best friend,' said another. Of course, you'll always find some people who'll tell you how hard it gets (one twin mum sent me a text message which said: 'Enjoy this quiet time,' which, to me, felt like it had a slightly smug 'just you wait' vibe to it).

There are challenges to come, but I truly believe that once you've got through the fourth trimester with twins, you've usually jumped over the hardest hurdle. As the next few months progress, you'll start to feel more like yourself, your hormones will settle down and you'll get into the swing of everything that caring for twin babies involves.

Looking ahead to the next few months, here are some of the hazards you'll face (but none of them are insurmountable!).

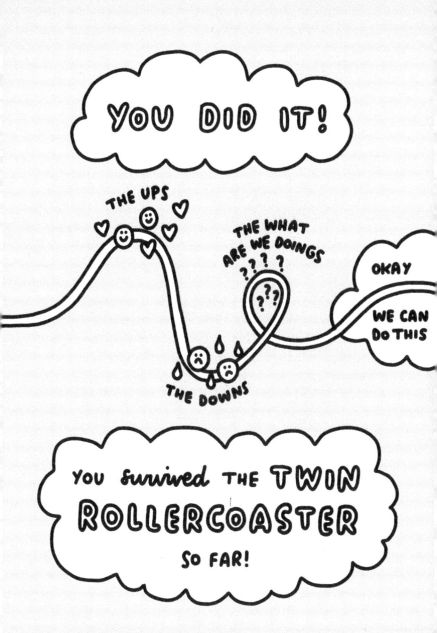

Weaning

The thought of weaning two babies at the same time filled me with dread. Some people love introducing their baby to food, but I just find it stressful. *What if they choke? What if they refuse all food? What if one baby eats well and the other doesn't?*

And the organisation needed is enough to make my head spin. 'I feel like I've only just got my head around breastfeeding and we're in a good rhythm, and now we have to think about *food*,' I wailed to my husband. When they turned six months, I went to the library and got a book on weaning and followed some useful accounts on Instagram – @sr_nutrition and @weanin15 – to give me tips and ideas on food. On their advice, we started the twins off with puréed green veg and bits of broccoli and green beans – doing a mix of baby-led (where you give finger-sized pieces of food to them to suck and chew on) and traditional purée weaning. Doing a mix felt like the right thing to do, for us. I liked giving them the ability to pick food up and choose to nibble on it, as well as giving them 'easier' puréed food to fill them up. It seemed to work for us, and before long, our twins were enthusiastically munching on salmon, scrambled egg, pasta Bolognese and mild chicken curry.

The good thing about weaning twins is that they see each other eating and it encourages them to try stuff. We went through a period of having their highchairs facing each other so that they could see their twin munching away.

The flipside of this, of course, is if one twin starts throwing food on the floor and clamping their mouth shut when the spoon comes their way, the other twin might follow suit!

My weaning tips

❋ Don't stress if most of the food ends up on the floor to start with.

❋ Start off with more bitter green veg before you introduce fruit and sweeter veg like carrot and squash.

❋ Put music on when they eat, to set the mood and give them the cue that it's eating time. We used to put soothing classical music on, but now we put Mother Goose Club songs on Spotify, or the digital station Fun Kids Junior, which has nursery rhymes that we can sing along to while they eat.

'A cheap shower curtain saved us from the mess!'

KIM, MUM TO BOY/GIRL TWINS, 19 MONTHS OLD

———————————

Oh my goodness! Weaning terrified and excited me all at once! My health visitor strongly encouraged me to do baby-led weaning, but I just couldn't face the mess. It didn't make sense to me – as adults we don't eat our food with our hands so why would you want to encourage your kids to do it?! She did give me one piece of excellent advice though, and that was to buy a cheap shower curtain and put it down under the high chairs. It has 100 per cent saved our carpet!

We started weaning when they turned six months old. A few weeks earlier, I'd been worried they wouldn't be ready at six months, especially as they were six weeks premature. But they suddenly started showing an interest and we went for it. We started with baby rice, then quickly moved onto puréed veg. We did a good two weeks of this before introducing fruit so that they didn't get too much of a sweet tooth. My girl twin took to weaning well and showed enthusiasm for pretty much everything. My boy would willingly open his mouth and try it, but everything (except sweet potato) was quickly followed with a grimace and spat out. At about eight ot nine months he got it though, and he eats well now. They seem to prefer facing each other in their high chairs rather than being side by side – I guess they find each other more interesting than me – and it seemed to end up with more being eaten than when they were side by side.

Going back to work

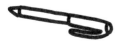

The decision to go back to work can be a real emotional crunch point for many twin mums. After spending your maternity leave getting to know these two little humans, you're suddenly looking at childcare options and spending less time with them. I went back to work fairly early after having my twins – when they were five months old – but that's because I work from home and our childcare was my husband! A primary-school teacher by trade, he stopped working just before the twins were born and became a stay-at-home dad. For us, this was the best option financially but we also took it knowing that I might need some extra emotional support in the early days, thanks to having a history of postnatal depression.

So when the time came, I started taking myself off to quiet rooms in the house to work, or popping to a coffee shop with my laptop. I felt incredibly lucky that I could duck my head in to see the twins during a work break. It was a far cry from when my eldest was a baby and I went back to working in an office. That first day of leaving her at nursery for a settling in session was so hard – I'm not sure who cried more, me or her. Before long, though, my daughter loved it – in fact she preferred being at nursery to being at home – and was hugely benefiting from socialising with lots of other little ones.

But as hard as the transition is, from being your twins' primary caregiver to being part-time, and going back to work, it's (thankfully) only a temporary stage. It gets so much easier for you, and them, as you all get used to the new situation.

'I'm so much happier working part-time'

KATHARINE, MUM TO ONE-YEAR-OLD TWINS
AND A THREE-YEAR-OLD SINGLETON

I went back to work when my twins were nine months old – I'm a freelance digital journalist and it felt like the right time to be going back to work. My eldest son, Ollie, was at preschool and we wanted to keep him there with all of his buddies, but I wasn't keen on putting the twins into nursery at such a young age. So we decided to get a nanny for three days a week – I felt happier that they'd be getting more dedicated childcare from her than a nursery. On the first day that she started, I stuck around to show her where everything was, and then ducked off, but I was an emotional wreck. I met a friend for coffee and told her that I wasn't sure I was doing the right thing.

As a freelancer, I needed to build my work up again, meet people, arrange work, so I wasn't that busy to start with and I felt so guilty that I was spending time away from the boys but not technically 'working'.

The first week was hard but the boys very quickly settled with the nanny and we haven't looked back. I'm definitely happier working part of the week and spending the rest of the week with the boys. It's good to have a bit of time to be 'me' and to use my brain in a different way. But the boys are still so small and I don't want to miss any special moments. I think we'll put them into nursery when they're a bit older but for now, having the nanny really works for us.

My tip is to try not to go headfirst into full-on work as soon as your childcare is sorted. If you can, give yourself some time to yourself. Looking after two babies is intense and physically and mentally exhausting. If you can afford to have a week off before starting work, try to dedicate some time to seeing friends, napping, going to the cinema or shopping. Once you start work, life will be exhausting in another way and you won't get this time again.

My getting back to work tips

✳ Think about what childcare option works best for you - a childminder might work out cheaper for two babies than a nursery.

✳ Consider (if you can) starting with one day a week of childcare and then increasing it, to ease everyone in gently.

✳ Remember that when they turn two, they might be able to go to a preschool, which is often cheaper than private nurseries and often run for half a day. And when they turn three, they get 30 hours of free childcare, which can go a long way!

Treating your twins as individuals

We've always found it easy to treat our twins as individuals because they're so different. There's no danger that we'd ever assume they have the same needs (just like they don't have the same needs as our eldest does!). In fact, they're so different that, despite us being told at our 12-week scan (see page 12) that we were expecting monochorionic identical twins, we think . . . (dramatic pause – big reveal coming) . . . that they actually must be non-identical. One has brown eyes; one has blue eyes. They have totally different facial features. One has short hair; one has long hair. We may get them DNA tested in the future, but for now, I'm assuming that when I was pregnant their two placentas fused and made it look like one placenta. So we have no difficulties treating them as individuals! One thing I do struggle with is not comparing their development. One twin rolled much earlier. The other crawled much sooner. One currently says no words, the other says around five or six words. It can be tempting to benchmark them against each other, but try not to.

My tips for treating your twins like individuals

❋ Dressing your twins differently can help you treat them as individuals.

❋ If you have non-identical twins, remember that there's nothing to say they should reach key milestones at the same time.

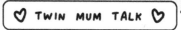

♡ TWIN MUM TALK ♡

'My twins have perfected the knack of going in opposite directions!'

BETH, MUM TO SEVEN-YEAR-OLD IDENTICAL TWIN GIRLS

As soon as your twins are on the go, your life becomes one big risk assessment. You are constantly having to evaluate which one is in more danger and you run to them first! My twins seemed to perfect the knack of always going in opposite directions, but I would advise that a playpen of some sort is a good idea, as well as also making sure they have an accident-free zone where they can play. This means that you can sit down and enjoy a quick drink in peace. My lounge quickly resembled a soft-play area, but it meant that I knew they were safe when I popped to the loo or made their lunch.

When out and about, I found reins useful, as it gave them some sort of freedom, but often I did feel like I was walking a bunch of cats on a lead! I tended to keep them in the pushchair for as long as possible until I knew there was a safe area for them to run off steam. I am a big fan of doing whatever makes your life easier and following your gut.

Just remember that they are your babies and people with one child often don't understand how challenging it can be, so you do what works for you!

'How I make sure my identical twins discover their own identities'

FIONA, MUM OF A FIVE-YEAR-OLD DAUGHTER
AND IDENTICAL TWIN BOYS, AGED THREE

———————

As an identical twin myself, I know how important it is to retain your own identity whilst also being part of a complex sibling relationship. Since their birth I have always dressed my second twin in stripes. It might just be a pair of socks but he always has stripes on. That way, family members know immediately which twin is which and there isn't any embarrassment on their part. It also means that I can look back on baby photos and I know which twin is which. My mum didn't know who was who with our baby photos because we were always dressed alike so I was keen not to put myself in the same situation.

My twins go to nursery at different times – one goes in the mornings and the other goes in the afternoons and it means they have much needed time apart and a chance to grow their own friendships. When they regroup at the end of the day they are genuinely pleased to see each other. They also have completely different friends at nursery, and their different personalities have been noticed and encouraged.

When they get on the move

'Just you wait until they're crawling!' If I had £10 for every time I heard this . . . But yes, your twins being able to move is a bit of a daunting prospect. Two crawling babies going in opposite directions can be tricky to manage, but it's not the big stress that many imagine it to be. When they're little and crawling it's easy enough to scoop one up and then scoop the other up. They can't crawl faster than you can run!

We created a little sectioned-off play area in our kitchen, with play mats and toys, which gave our twins a decent amount of space to crawl around in, but we could close the stair gate and keep them safe while we cooked dinner or dashed to the door to answer it. We do sometimes have to have eyes in the back of our heads – we might be reading with one twin and then notice that the other twin has clambered onto the sofa and has opened a pot of Sudocrem that she discovered.

My crawling tips

❋ Stairgates and large play pens are a godsend for keeping your crawling twins safe. They're useful for parents of singletons but for a twin parent they're essential. It's surprising how quickly two crawling or toddling babies can be out of the room and causing mayhem before you even notice!

❋ If you have friends on maternity leave who are stay-at-home parents or who work part-time, ask if they'll come along with you to a playgroup. Even if they have their own little one to bring, two pairs of eyes on three babies is easier than just you chasing after two!

When they fight for your attention

When my twins were really small, having them both cry at the same time was a fairly stressful situation. But as they get older, they fight for my attention in a different way. I'll be sitting with one on my knee and the other will crawl up and wedge herself in between me and her sister! It'll usually end in tears as the twin being shoved out of the way (understandably) protests and complains. Keeping both of them happy when they both want my full attention at the same time can be a challenge. Now that they're starting to understand instructions, I've started talking about taking turns and sharing (but let's be honest, it takes a long time for little ones to understand this concept, doesn't it?!).

My tips for keeping both twins happy

★ Any time you can have one-to-one time with one of your twins, take it. It's so lovely to just sit with one of them and play or chat to them, and it (theoretically and hopefully!) means they'll be less demanding of your attention when their twin is around.

★ Just accept that there will be times when they tussle for your attention and often it varies depending on their personality. I have one twin who (I suspect) thinks she 'owns' me and is very cross if her sister tries to sit on my knee. The other one is much more chilled and doesn't seem to mind either way.

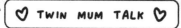

♡ TWIN MUM TALK ♡

'My twins are used to sharing attention – but that doesn't stop them complaining!'

ISABEL, MUM TO 17-MONTH OLD NON-IDENTICAL TWINS
AND A THREE-YEAR-OLD SINGLETON

———

At 17 months, my twins are already using the language 'my turn'. They know that they sometimes have to wait for individual attention but this doesn't stop them complaining! I have to say though, my singleton child was the same. I guess to a certain extent, toddlers will be toddlers and when they want something they definitely let you know about it!

I think twins are very used to sharing attention though, as it's what they've always known, so in some ways my twins find it easier than my older son does. We try to make a conscious effort to make time for each of our children individually. We've found that the twins actually seem to prefer being together. When they're taken out separately they are a bit freaked out and anxious. They ask where their twin is a lot, so for now we spend a lot of family time together.

We use coloured sand timers of three minutes and five minutes to help the twins manage turn taking and them wanting adult attention. We found this visual tool can help support their understanding that they will have their turn and it gives them something to focus on whilst they wait. My son, who is three, now uses the timers independently when he wants a toy that one of the twins is playing with. I hope in time the twins will also begin to use this strategy to self-manage their sharing.

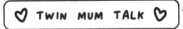

♡ TWIN MUM TALK ♡

'I took my baby twins backpacking!'

SHELLIE, MUM TO TODDLER TWINS, AGED 25 MONTHS

'Backpacking with baby twins? You must be either brave or stupid!' was the usual response when we told people about our summer plans to travel around Poland and Belarus with one-year-old twins. But we'd been backpackers before the twins arrived and the small detail of baby twins wasn't going to stop us. We live in Spain, which means we'd already flown at least five times with the twins when going back to visit family, each time learning something new and tweaking our travel style.

Envisaging the journey before can help. Run it all through in your mind from the moment you step out of your front door until the moment you're collected on the other side. You can run through any possible problems and troubleshoot them in advance. You can imagine the journey going positively and then during the actual journey, channel that feeling of, 'I bloody bossed the imaginary run through so I can boss this too'. Compartmentalising the journey is also a great way to help yourself: house to airport phase one. Through security phase two etc. We check our pram in at the desk and dismantle it into a pram suitcase, which means we can squeeze a few extras in the space around it. We then carry the twins in a sling each.

I highly recommend buying a pram bag, it was one of our best purchases. My tip is to pack two backpacks with the same stuff, in case you are separated, and smile at everyone you pass – the baggage handlers, the security person, the check in assistant, the airline steward, the pilot . . . everyone.

Going on holiday

We haven't braved travelling abroad with our twins yet. There just seems to be so much to think about – timing flights with naps, keeping them occupied on the flight, car seats on airport transfers, double buggies that are compact enough for travel, finding accommodation for a family of five . . . it makes my head spin! So we did two UK breaks in the first year of having our twins around – Center Parcs with their grandparents and then a lodge holiday in Cornwall. We still had to be a bit more organised than usual – planning the car journey stops to feed the babies and change nappies, and buying travel cots and blackout blinds to ensure the twins would sleep. I remember worrying that they wouldn't settle in a room they were unfamiliar with (they did!).

My travelling with twins tips:

* Wait until you're comfortable with the idea of going on holiday with your twins. There's no pressure and if the idea stresses you out, do some day trips first to get you used to going further afield with them.

* Caravans, lodges and Airbnbs can be a great idea for families with twins as you have more flexibility on bedrooms and sleeping arrangements (and if you get your twins to nap/sleep then you can hang out in the living room while they sleep in the bedroom – if you're in one hotel room, you have to sit in the dark!).

* Check what's available at the accommodation you've booked. We booked a lodge with two cots, but on arrival discovered it didn't include mattresses or sheets!

Potty training

I wish I could share some brilliant words of wisdom with you about potty-training twins but my twins aren't even two yet, so potty training is a long way off. What I will say, though, is that we left potty training our older daughter until quite late – she just didn't seem ready, so we didn't ever push it. So when we did potty train her, she went straight to the loo! And I think we only had one 'accident' because she was really ready and being older, really got the concept of recognising the need to go and telling us.
Since I'm not able to offer any advice, I've asked potty-training expert and author of *Potty Training Magic* to share her top tips for twin parents...

How to potty train twins

Amanda Jenner, potty training expert (@pottytrainingacademy)

BE READY TO POTTY TRAIN YOUR TWINS AT DIFFERENT TIMES

A lot of parents want to potty train twins at the same time but twins are two individuals and they may be developing at a different rate.

LOOK OUT FOR SIGNS FROM EACH TWIN THAT THEY MIGHT BE READY

Those signs might be one of the twins stopping in their tracks when they're doing a wee or poo, noticing what they're doing, being familiar with them soiling themselves. It helps if you refer to their bodily functions and show an interest and then insist on changing them when they've soiled. Read them both potty-training books and show them flash cards.

DON'T WAIT UNTIL THEY'RE BOTH READY

One of them might show an interest and the other might

show none at all. But I would definitely go ahead with potty training the twin that is showing an interest. If you wait until they're both ready, you might have missed your window with one of them!

ONCE YOU'RE POTTY TRAINING ONE TWIN, IT MIGHT ENCOURAGE THE OTHER

Often what happens is when you start potty training one, the other might become inquisitive and try to follow their twin. It's not always the case but gradually they might start to show signs that they're ready too.

BUY TWO POTTIES AND LET THEM PICK ONE OUT

If you buy one potty, you might find they'll fight over it. You may have one twin using the potty and the other twin comes along and says they need a wee! Let your twins choose their potties – they might want the same colour or design, but they might want something different. It helps for them to have 'their' potty and they've got to like what they're going to use.

USE REWARD CHARTS BUT DON'T COMPARE THEIR PROGRESS

I'd recommend buying or making two reward charts with each twin's name on top, so they know which one is theirs. You might find one twin is more competitive than the other which spurs on the other. It's not a race but they are individuals so it's important to reward them as individuals. Don't compare them though! Don't tell one twin that the other one is doing better. The language you use around little children when potty training is important – use positive language and be careful not to talk negatively about them and their potty-training progress to others in front of them – they listen to everything you say and it can affect their progress.

'*I potty-trained my twins at two different times!*'

MELANIE, MUM TO TWO-YEAR-OLD NON-IDENTICAL TWINS

———————

When I decided the time was right to start potty training my twin boys it felt like one of the last early motherhood hurdles, the next thing I needed to pass and if I could crack it then I would have ticked off another big milestone. I decided to potty train Toby first – he was two years and five months. I started with Ollie a month later, so he was around two years and six months.

I thought they were ready because I noticed they'd started to tell me when they had done something in their nappy and they would also get frustrated and ask for a clean nappy even if it wasn't that full. I started to put them on the toilet in the morning and before the bath and they got on with this really well so it made me think they may be ready.

I decided to potty train them at different times – firstly because Toby was showing all the signs I mentioned before Ollie and would regularly sit on the potty I kept around, but Ollie not so much. He just didn't seem as interested. I really didn't want to push him or rush anything. They are different in so many ways, I always thought they would be ready at different times. But also, I wasn't actually sure I was ready to be doing them both at the same time! It felt like a lot to take on at once.

It did take me some time to crack it and it wasn't quite the smooth, easy ride I was hoping for. We've had a few moments of them both having accidents on the floor and there being tears and screaming! I think as a mum when we start something like potty training it becomes a bit of a personal project, so when it doesn't go as we planned we somehow feel like we have failed. But trust me, however it goes or however long it takes, they are toddlers and toddlers are unpredictable at the best of times!

My advice would be that although they are twins every child is different and they may be ready and get there at different times and that's OK. Try not to compare them. Twins are naturally quite competitive so you will likely find if you start one the other will watch and want to be involved, which is actually very helpful. Don't ever feel pressured to start one because the other seems ready, starting with just one of them is fine and to start early will only bring stress. When they are really ready it will be much easier and quicker. Let them pick a potty each and some fun pants and generally keep talking about it and how totally amazing they are, praise really is everything!

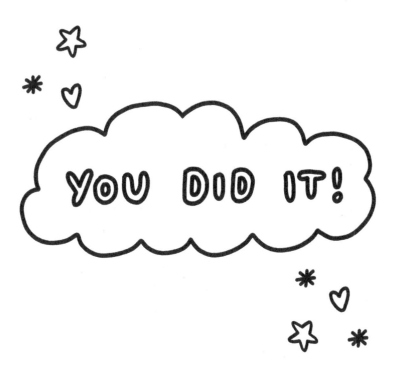

One final word . . .

Having twins is – undoubtedly – an emotional roller coaster. But you can ride the downs as well as the ups. There are days when it all feels really hard. But then there are days when it seems a bit easier, and that feeling you get when you have totally nailed a day with your twins, is second to none!

It's such a cliché but life with twins does get easier. We've covered the first few months here because it's the most emotionally challenging time. Yes, there are challenges ahead, but as your hormones settle and as you start to reclaim a bit more of 'you', everything will feel a bit easier.

They say practice makes perfect – the more you do this stuff, the easier it feels. The things that you struggled with in these early days? You'll look back on them and wonder why it felt so hard. You'll be changing two nappies with your eyes closed, one-handed, while dictating a shopping list to Siri. I promise!

And – another cliché incoming – twins might be double the work, but they're also double the joy. The smiles you'll get, the giggles, the cuddles. Twice over! It's such a special, special thing. So while you're surviving the early days of twin motherhood, pause and take a moment to reflect on how far you've come. From that moment you found out it was twins, through your pregnancy, giving birth and through to today. What an incredible achievement!

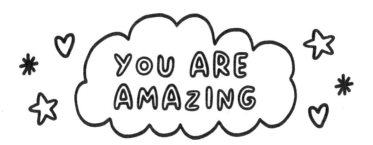

YOU ARE AMAZING

THE BEST THING ABOUT having twins IS:

....

....

....

THE MOST CHALLENGING
THING ABOUT having twins IS:

....

....

....

THE MOST SURPRISING
THING ABOUT having twins IS:

....

....

....

Resources

Twins Trust (formerly TAMBA)
twinstrust.org

NHS Twins information
www.nhs.uk/conditions/
pregnancy-and-baby/giving-
birth-to-twins

Homestart
www.home-start.org.uk

Gingerbread
www.gingerbread.org.uk

Doula UK
doula.org.uk

Neighbourhood Doulas
www.neighbourhooddoulas.org

Positive Birth Company
thepositivebirthcompany.co.uk

The Lullaby Trust
www.lullabytrust.org.uk

Squeezy app
www.squeezyapp.com

Mumsnet
Mumsnet.com

The Motherload
facebook.com/groups/
wearethemotherload

**BCLC breastfeeding
counsellors**
lcgb.org/find-an-ibclc

Mind's 'Mums Matter' service
www.mind.org.uk/information-
support/mums-matter

***The Little Book of Self-Care
for New Mums***
available in bookshops

Index

With thanks to . . .

A huge thank you to everyone involved with this book. To everyone at Vermilion: Sam Jackson for giving me the opportunity to turn my book dreams into a reality, brilliant editors Emma Owen, Leah Feltham, Justine Taylor and Lindsay Kaubi, plus all the people behind the scenes who worked their magic! Massive thanks to Nikki Dupin and Emma Wells at studio Nic&Lou for the amazing colourful book cover. It just sums me up perfectly and is exactly how I imagined my book would look. Thank you to the hugely talented Veronica Dearly, who illustrated the book with her incredible drawings. Thank you to both Zoe King and Rebecca Ritchie at AM Heath for being fabulous agents. For holding my hand when I needed it and for believing that I can do this!

I'm so grateful to the women who allowed me to interview them for this book; all of the mothers who shared their experiences and those who contributed their expert knowledge and wisdom. Thank you to you all. Thank you to the friends who kept me sane while I wrote this book: Molly, Em, Emily (and to Sarah for that pep-talk phone call when I was deep in imposter syndrome!) and all the school mums who were ready with Prosecco. Thank you to Vickie and Deborah, whose introductions in the publishing world kick-started it all.

Last (but not least) thank you to Mr P who gives me so much encouragement and who held the fort at home while I spent evenings and weekends writing this book, in what was an already challenging 2020. You're awesome.

Alison Perry is a journalist and mum of twins (and an older daughter). She is an award-winning blogger with her site Not Another Mummy Blog (notanothermummyblog. com) and also hosts *Not Another Mummy Podcast* where she has chatted to guests such as Philippa Perry, Meg Mathews and Emma Bunton. She lives in London and you can find her on Instagram **@iamalisonperry**